FOLK REMEDIES
HEALING WISDOM

Writers

Paul Bergner

David J. Hufford, Ph.D.

Consultant

Ara Der Marderosian, Ph.D.

Illustrator

John Zielinski

Publications International, Ltd.

All rights reserved under International and Pan American copyright conventions. Copyright © 1998 Publications International, Ltd. This publication may not be reproduced or quoted in whole or in part by any means whatsoever without written permission from:

Louis Weber, C.E.O.
Publications International, Ltd.
7373 North Cicero Avenue
Lincolnwood, Illinois 60646

Permission is never granted for commercial purposes.

Printed in U.S.A.

Photo credits:

Front cover: **Archive Photos** (bottom); **Quilt by Joan M. Rigal/Siede Preis Photography (background).**

Back cover: **Quilt by Joan M. Rigal/Siede Preis Photography**

Interior photos: **FPG International:** Steve Belkowitz: 348; Ernest Manewal: 137; **Dario Perla/International Stock:** 48; **SuperStock:** 46.

NOTE: Neither the Editors of Consumer Guide™ and Publications International, Ltd., nor the authors, consultants, editors, or publisher take responsibility for any possible consequence from any treatment, procedure, exercise, dietary modification, action, or application of medication or preparation by any person reading or following the information in this book. The publication of this book does not constitute the practice of medicine, and this book does not attempt to replace your physician or your pharmacist. Before undertaking any course of treatment, the authors, consultants, editors, and publisher advise the reader to check with a physician or other health care provider.

Ara Der Marderosian, Ph.D., is professor of Pharmacognosy and Medicinal Chemistry and is Roth Chair of Natural Products at Philadelphia College of Pharmacy & Science. He has researched extensively in the areas of medicinal and poisonous plants, folkloric medicinal plants, hallucinogenic botanicals, herbal teas, ginseng, and medical foods.

Paul Bergner (Remedies) is editor of *Medical Herbalism* and is clinic director at the Rocky Mountain Center for Botanical Studies. He has published *The Naturopathic Physician* and *Clinical Nutrition Update* magazines and has written many books, including *The Healing Power of Minerals and Trace Elements* and *The Healing Power of Echinacea, Goldenseal, and the Immune System Herbs.*

David J. Hufford, Ph.D. (Introduction and Special Interests) is director of The Doctors Kienle Center for Humanistic Medicine and Academic Director of the Medical Ethnography Collection at Pennsylvania State University, College of Medicine. He also is professor of Medical Humanities, Behavioral Science, and Family & Community Medicine. Dr. Hufford serves on the editorial boards of several journals, including *Alternative Therapies in Health & Medicine.*

Additional contributing writers:

Alexandra F. Griswold, Ph.D., instructor, Department of Folklore and Folklife at the University of Pennsylvania

Bonnie O'Connor, Ph.D., professor, Community & Preventive Medicine, Medical College of Pennsylvania

Barbara Rieti, Ph.D., writer and researcher in the field of folklore

Joan L. Saverino, Ph.D., instructor, Department of Folklore and Folklife at the University of Pennsylvania

Editorial assistance: Gloria Bucco, president, Gloria Bucco & Associates

Contributing illustrator: Dan Krovatin

❦ Contents ❦

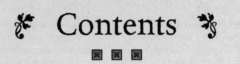

CONTENTS

Special Interests

Defining Folk Medicine

"Folklore" is the traditional knowledge of ordinary people. Folk medicine, one kind of folklore, is made up of the ideas and practices of ordinary people concerning health and illness. In saying that folklore is "traditional," we emphasize that it has lasted through time—that it was not "born yesterday." But there is no hard and fast rule about how old something must be to be "folk." The jump rope rhymes of today's children—one kind of folklore—include some elements that are centuries old and others that have been newly created by the children who are using them. The same is true of folk medicine. Some of the remedies found in oral tradition in the United States today are truly ancient, such as the idea that health is influenced by heat and cold (as in the folk belief that getting chilled can cause one to "catch" a cold). Other items of contemporary folk medicine are quite new—for example, the odd belief that radon gas (produced by the decay of radium) is a remedy for lung ailments! This colorless and odorless gas has only been known since 1900, and its use as a health remedy has involved sitting in abandoned uranium mines. Of course, what is odd about this belief is that radon gas is actually a cause of lung cancer. So, the belief in radon as a remedy is not only recent—it is dangerous! However, this example is not meant to suggest that folk medicine is generally useless—far from it, as we shall see.

Folklore includes a great variety of culture, from proverbs to quilt designs and from folktales to folk songs, as well as folk medicine. What all folklore has in common is that it is the property of ordinary people—that is, people who are not "officially" recognized as experts. For this reason, folklore tends to be passed on by word of mouth—what folklorists call "oral tradition." So while "classical" music is taught in music appreciation class, folk songs are learned from those around us. (We learned to sing "Happy Birthday to You.") Official "bio-medicine" is taught in medical schools and passed on to the public by physicians— from the Surgeon General on down to your family doctor. Folk medicine is learned from parents and friends or provided by community folk practitioners. It would be a mistake to imagine that the boundaries between these forms of culture are always so clear and sharp. What is the difference between the folk medicine actually collected from oral tradition and the old "regular medicine" from the last century? And what about the medical traditions of other cultures?

In folk medicine, as in language, religion, and all areas of culture, "purity" is rare. Culture develops through a mixing process, and the persistence of folk medicine and other kinds of folklore through the centuries demonstrates that, while this mixing does not always destroy traditions, it does constantly change them. In folk medicine what we see are trends, not absolutes. At the same time, it must be granted that the folk medicine traditions of people (for example, the American Indians) whose culture has been placed under great pressure by modern circumstances is sometimes threatened with being lost or changed beyond recognition.

Many people can respect most folklore—even if it is not from a tradition they identify with or actually appreciate. However, many do not have the same attitude toward folk medicine. Because folk belief is made up of things believed by ordinary people to be true, as opposed to what experts teach us to be true, it is often assumed that folk belief is mere superstition or false belief. Fortunately, in recent years, most people have begun to reconsider this attitude. After all, even the experts can be wrong. Folk medicine is very closely related to peoples' experience with their bodies and their minds and the world around them, and that experience is generally worth paying attention to! No one is an expert on your experience except you! Of course, as the "radon remedy" illustrates, ordinary people are sometimes wrong in ways that only an expert can best explain. Today, we are beginning to see more of a balance in the ways that we evaluate both expert and folk ideas concerning health.

THE HISTORY OF MEDICINE

Because of the great practical importance of medical beliefs and practices—both official and folk—we'll start with the related issues of efficacy, risk, and quackery. What reasons might we have to believe that some folk medicine "really works" and some does not? What risks may be associated with using folk medicine?

Official medicine generally assumes that it has accepted, or is in the process of accepting, every healing practice that has been shown to be effective. Medical history has always been intimately associated with folk medicine, and today official medicine actually defines folk and alternative medicines by exclusion. This dominant position of official medicine is a very new thing in Western culture. So we must begin with a little medical history.

Before the 20th century, the licensing of physicians was largely honorific, and

it did not exclude unli-
censed healers from prac-
tice. In 1760, New York
City passed the first law
for examining and exclu-
sively licensing doctors,
but that law was never
enforced. In 1763, the
physicians of Norwich,
Connecticut, asked the
colonial legislature for
licensing "to distinguish
between Honest and Inge-
nious physicians and the
Quack or Empirical Pre-
tender." The problem of
competition was recog-
nized as serious, but the
request was denied. Fol-
lowing the American Revo-
lution, medical societies
organized and legislatures
granted licensing, but these
laws were powerless and
ineffective. Americans
have always been a fiercely
independent lot, and the
high value placed on individual choice was in direct
conflict with the desire of
medical professionals to
control health care. As a
result, folk medicine and a
variety of popular forms of
alternative medicine flour-
ished openly. In fact, if we
had been there in the
mid-century, we would
have had a hard time
knowing just which practitioners were considered to
be "regular" and which
were "alternative."

Medical schools were,
by and large, small busi-
nesses, and the quality of
their graduates was very
unreliable. Harvard was
among the first of the
medical schools to attempt
reform. In 1869, Charles
Eliot, the president of
Harvard, said, "The igno-
rance and general incom-
petency of the average
graduate of American
Medical schools, at the
time when he [is turned]
loose upon the commu-
nity, is something horrible
to contemplate." Both the
nature of the competition
and the quality of medical
education changed dra-
matically after Abraham
Flexner, a young educator
with a B.A. degree from
Johns Hopkins, carried out
a study of medical schools.
Flexner made surprise
visits to the schools and
documented the often
pathetic resources in
laboratories, the lack of

access to patients, the incompetent faculty, and the generally disreputable state of most American medical schools. His report, published in 1910, recommended that 100 of the 131 existing medical schools be closed, although 70 eventually survived. Flexner did not start the reform movement in medical education, but his report was a watershed event in the transformation of medicine. However, that reform not only improved the basics of education for "regular physicians," it also established a principle that many expected would eradicate the competition—including folk medicine. A whole new medicine, organized around "regular medicine" was to replace all separate medical sects.

The new medicine was to be objective and scientific. It was assumed that would mean that all treatments shown to work would be included and all those that were ineffective would be excluded. The Pure Food and Drug Act of 1906 and medical licensure soon consolidated the medical profession's political power. Using that power the profession actively worked to prevent others from practicing medicine without a license. Doctors labeled those who did not fit the medical model as "quacks," and their efforts to eradicate quackery were presented as public education and protection.

The word "quack" comes from the old Dutch word "quacksalver." The term became popular in the 1500s and described people who sold salves and ointments—and who generally made exaggerated claims for them. Some have suggested that the word is also derived in part from quicksilver, which is the element mercury. Mercury was a common ingredient in regular medicines of the day as well as in the home remedies sold by quacks.

By the 20th century, the term quack was not at all restricted to ointment sellers. Modern dictionary definitions are very specific about what the word means: people who pretend to have medical knowledge that they do not in fact have. Unfortunately, the term is used very loosely, so that it is often applied to all sorts of healers whose practices were believed to be ineffective. This sloppy use of the word merely serves to insult those with whom conventional medicine disagrees. But still worse, it "gives cover" to the real medical frauds, of whom there are many. After all, with no distinction made between charlatans and sincere folk healers, it is much harder to identify the charlatans.

THE EFFECTIVENESS OF FOLK MEDICINE

It has been shown that some folk medicine works—in the medical sense, that is. What's more, folk medicine is capable of serving goals that are broader and more complicated than those of modern medicine. One recent example comes from women's folk health traditions. For many years, women have learned from other women that eating live culture yogurt helps to reduce vaginal yeast infections. In 1992, a study published in the *Annals of Internal Medicine* concluded that this practice is, in fact, effective. It is fascinating to consider that such a widely known and practiced element of folk medicine, used to treat a very common medical problem, could have been ignored by conventional medicine for so long. Even now, after this study, the use of this remedy has not become standard medical practice.

Prescription medications not only have their desired medical effects, but they also have side effects, some of which can be quite serious. The same is true for folk medicines. Many people have the mistaken idea that "If it's natural, it can't hurt me." Some of the most powerful poisons that we know of are found in nature. And every year, in addition to those individuals who are poisoned accidentally by plants, there are people who enter hospitals because plant remedies they prepared to treat medical conditions have in fact poisoned them. Poisoning can happen in several different ways.

Some plant medicines that are effective are simply too dangerous to use outside medical supervision. Some popular plants in folk medicine have turned out to cause health problems when used over time. Some plant medicines can become dangerous through adulteration. This can happen either by accident or intentionally. Accidents happen when someone gathering herbs in the wild unintentionally picks the wrong plant or happens to grab two plants at once, one intended and the other not noticed. Because many commercially available herbs come from outside the country and the products are not regulated, sometimes herbal

medicines contain enough plant poison to cause sickness or even death.

All three of these dangers are greatest for infants or very sick people with a low body weight. These dangers have been most frequently associated with commercially available herbal medicines. These risks are not enormous, but they are real. It seems prudent, therefore, to learn about plant medicine before you try herbal remedies.

FOLK MEDICINE AND SPIRITUALITY

In addition to herbs, folk medicine places a strong and consistent emphasis on spiritual matters, and many folk remedies involve rituals and prayers of various kinds. Some people call such practices "superstition." Some strongly religious people find the spirituality of folk medicine to be primitive or even wicked—for example, those whose tradition does not use ritual may find the religious rituals of folk medicine to be similar to "black magic." Others reject the spirituality of folk medicine as superstition because they reject all spiritual belief. These skeptics often say that belief in prayer and other spiritual activities is irrational because it lacks any possible evidence.

In 1988, a cardiologist named Randolph Byrd, M.D., published an article in the *Southern Medical Journal* in which he described a study that measured the effect of prayer on a large group of patients who had suffered heart attacks. Many psychologists and medical researchers over the years have shown that praying can powerfully affect those who do it, and this has generally been explained in terms of positive mental effects. But Byrd did not study people praying for themselves. He divided almost 400 patients into an experimental group and a control group. (Neither the participating patients nor their doctors and nurses had any way of knowing how the groups were divided.) Dr. Byrd gave the first names of the patients in the experimental group to people in prayer groups. Each prayer group had been in existence, praying for others, for a substantial period of time. The members of these groups agreed to pray regularly for the people who were assigned to them. In the end, Dr. Byrd found that the patients who received prayer did better than those who did not. They were not miraculously healed, but they recovered with fewer complications and setbacks, and this difference was highly significant statistically. Today, some medical researchers consider it proven that prayer can have a direct effect on health, while others do not. Additional studies have been undertaken to try to confirm Byrd's findings. At any rate, there is now some evidence for the efficacy of prayer.

FOLK MEDICINE AND CULTURAL AUTHORITY

Folk tradition has long existed in tension with official medicine. An important source of that tension, and a large part of the difference between the two, involves cultural authority. Cultural authority is the power to make statements about how the world works—about the real nature of the world—and have those statements accepted. Throughout history, in most parts of the world, it was life experience that gave people cultural authority. Religious status and a few other factors, such as the family into which a person was born, could also influence one's authority. In folk medicine, the knowledge of remedies is learned orally, representing the accumulated knowledge of past generations. Evaluation of the treatment is done by the patient's observations of what seems to help.

In the 19th century, as science and technology began the rapid change that now characterizes our modern world, the structure of cultural authority changed. Scientific discoveries increasingly revealed important but invisible things about the world, from invisibly small bacteria to radiation. It became more and more obvious that we could not know everything important about the world with unaided senses. Too many things you could not see might make you sick. As a result of this growing division between everyday experience and scientific knowledge, which was strongly supported by the apparent advantages that technology could deliver, modern society shifted. An unspoken agreement developed in which the experts in science and technology were given cultural authority and the right to govern their own institutions.

The internal control of experts over the definition of their own expertise includes the opportunity to set the limits on the area to which their expertise applies. The result is that the scope of expert cultural authority has grown consistently in modern society. Of course, that means that, at the same time, the scope of authority based on life experience, and not technical training, has decreased. The best medical care has come to be understood not as the accumulation of past wisdom but rather as the very latest technique, and the very latest technique is often explained in terms of how it puts past ideas to rest.

Up through the 1960s many believed that this social change in authority was irreversible and that technical knowledge would become the only kind of knowledge considered valid. But the 1960s brought deep change— ranging from the Hippie movement to the consumer movement, civil rights and women's liberation, even the Charismatic movement in Christian religion. All of these changes were rebellion against various kinds of authority and were a reassertion of the right of people to find, in their own experience, some valid basis for understanding and evaluating the world. The result has not been the complete overthrow of expert authority, but rather a process of trimming back that authority. In medicine, the idea of "informed consent," which requires doctors to tell patients what is proposed as treatment and why it is proposed, is an example of the reduction of medical authority and the return of some authority to the patient.

IN CLOSING

Most folk medicine traditions stress the underlying causes of disease as well as the immediate causes. The underlying causes are usually seen as some kind of imbalance or lack of harmony within the body. These causes range from sin to an improper balance of foods in the diet. A sick person may bear responsibility for the sickness, but it is also possible that the sickness is the result of someone else's wrongdoing. Folk medicine tends to have a strong moral tone, always trying to fix the blame for misfortune.

The moral element and the importance of harmony and balance are factors in folk medicine that lead to a sense of personal health's interconnectedness with the community, the physical environment, and the cosmos. This suggests a major function of all healing systems: the integration of the experience of sickness within a meaningful view of the world. Such an integration helps the sufferer to bring the maximum number of resources to bear on his illness and provides a rationale for efforts at prevention as well as treatment (such as protective amulets, blessings and pilgrimages, a good diet and exercise, and avoidance of poor social relations that could provoke witchcraft or the envy that leads to the evil eye). A rationale of this kind makes it possible to understand specific causes of disease on the basis of general principles, such as hot-cold balance or God's law. This complex, multi-causal view of disease etiology and appropriate treatments has often been called the "holistic outlook" of folk medicine. This view is usually quite open to modern medical knowledge. It accepts medical ideas of etiology: It is believed a germ can cause a disease, for example. But, in folk medicine, a germ causes disease in a particular person (at a particular time) for any number of reasons, including sinfulness, evil eye, poor diet, or because of decreased vital energy.

An emphasis on a special kind of "energy" that is unique to living things is almost universal in folk medical systems, and it is crucial in mediating the concepts of harmony, balance, and integration. This energy element places folk medicine within the tradition that, in Western thought, has been called vitalism. Vitalism says that life is made possible by a non-physical kind of force, often called vital energy (from *vita,* the Latin word for life). This energy is often believed to be distinct from the physical body that it animates and to be capable of a separate existence. The idea of human souls can be an example of this kind of energy. This concept of vitalism provides links among a great variety of specific theories of healing and general physical and metaphysical theories.

Folk healers often view their activities as a transfer of good energy to a patient and, often, the removal of negative energy. When working on the material level, as opposed to the spiritual level, Mexican-American *curanderos* manipulate positive energies and expel negative vibrating energies (called *vibraciones*) with incantations and certain material "tools." This is done to correct the patient's field of vital energy. Similar ideas about energy are very popular among modern alternative medical systems, such as chiropractic and homeopathy. (The commitment of these systems to the idea of a special vital energy is part of what has kept them "alternative.") Probably the most famous idea of vital energy in alternative medicine today is the Chinese concept of *chi.* This reference to the flow, transmission, and balance of life energies exists in folk medical traditions around the world and must certainly indicate the existence of some human universals in the perception of health, illness, and healing.

The complexity of these meanings illustrates another difference between folk and modern medicine: the variety of goals explicitly being served. The explicit goals of modern medicine can be briefly stated as the reducing of the harmful effects of disease. In most folk medical systems, this goal is found alongside a variety of non-medical goals; for example, assigning social responsibility for misfortune (as in witchcraft) and obtaining salvation in religious healing.

Finally, the techniques of folk medicine are almost entirely ones that are broadly legal, require little or no technology, and are therefore available to practically everyone. Although the highly learned healer generally has a body of knowledge that requires time and special circumstances to acquire, the individual elements are nonetheless generally available to all. Thus, the materials of these systems can readily be organized into all levels of health behavior—from first aid and home treatment to the most specialized and authoritative forms. This makes it very easy for people to enter folk medical systems. Folk medicine lacks many of the official barriers found in scientific medicine, and it makes available to patients a wide range of options for varying levels of personal involvement and decision making. For many patients, this is an attractive feature of folk medicine.

In the pages to come you will find a great variety of folk medical practices. Some of these practices will seem simple, such as drinking cranberry juice to reduce the risk of urinary tract infections. Others will seem outlandish and bizarre, including those folk remedies that require animal sacrifice! The remedies described in this book come from many different communities and represent the accumulated ideas and observations of centuries of healers. Like scientific medicine, some folk medicine is obsolete, some is dangerous, and some is ahead of its time. But all of these ideas represent the struggles of human communities to make sense of disease, suffering, and death and to do something about the human condition.

—David Hufford, Ph.D.

Allergies, Hives, and Hay Fever

Our bodies are constantly assaulted by substances from the environment, in the form of bacteria, viruses, molds, dust, pollen, and other potential invaders. Our immune system reacts to these substances through chemical and blood responses that attempt to neutralize the invaders or eliminate them from the body. One specialized immune response is the allergic reaction, in which specialized cells stimulated by an invading substance release the chemical histamine into the tissues. The histamine can cause swelling, increased circulation, and sneezing, actions designed to isolate the invader, eliminate it, or render it harmless. An allergic reaction can occur in the respiratory tract, digestive tract, skin, or eyes.

An allergic reaction is a healthy, protective response to an invader, but, in some individuals, the body overreacts, and the uncomfortable reactions are far in excess of what is necessary to neutralize the offending substance. The most noticeable allergic symptoms are sneezing, red swollen eyes, shortness of breath (in asthma), rashes, eczema, or the swelling that accompanies insect bites and stings. Food allergies can also cause symptoms in the digestive tract, but these are usually less noticeable to the sufferer than the external reactions above. The worst type of allergic reaction—called anaphylaxis—is an overwhelming allergic reaction that can lead to death. Any swelling of the airways or shortness of breath during an allergic reaction is a medical emergency.

Allergies tend to run in families, so some people may be genetically predisposed to having them. It has also been suggested that nutrient deficiencies common in the modern diet may also contribute to allergies. Dietary deficiencies of calcium and magnesium, which are common deficiencies in Americans, can also increase allergic symptoms. Studies have shown that the body's stores of vitamin C correlate inversely with the release of histamine during an allergy attack, so an abundant dietary intake of vitamin C may reduce allergy symptoms. Omega-3 essential fatty acids, such as occur naturally in cold-water fish and wild game, are also natural anti-inflammatory substances that can reduce the intensity of allergies.

Antihistamine drugs and avoidance of allergens are the most common conventional treatments for symptoms of allergy. The drugs work by blocking the effects of histamine in the tissues, but they do not reduce its release. Desensitization involves medical treatments where small amounts of an allergen may also be injected into the body in the form of allergy shots in order to reduce the body's reaction to it.

The folk remedies listed here do not address the cause of allergies but may reduce allergy symptoms through their astringent or anti-inflammatory actions. Also, avoid herbal remedies that are made up of flower parts (such as chamomile and echinacea) because these contain allergic pollen.

Remedies

ALLERGIES AND HAY FEVER

HORSERADISH: Horseradish (*Armoracia rusticana*), popular today as a sushi condiment, was an early American folk remedy for hay fever. If you've used it as a condiment, you're probably well aware that it causes watery eyes and a burning sensation in the sinus tissues. These effects are due to its constituent allyl-isothiocyanate, which is related chemically to the substances in watercress, red radish, and brown and yellow mustard. Scientific studies have shown that allyl-isothiocyanate has decongestant and anti-asthmatic properties.

☞ DIRECTIONS: Purchase grated horseradish as a condiment. Take a dose of ¼ teaspoon during a congestive hay fever attack. You can take horseradish as often as desired—or as much as you can stand!

An alternate method, if you have access to fresh horseradish root, comes from an old New England remedy. Take fresh horseradish roots, wash, and blend, skin and all, in your blender. Fill half of a 1-quart jar with the ground roots. Add enough vinegar to cover the roots, and close the jar tightly. Store the jar at room temperature. When suffering a hay fever attack, remove the cap, place your nose into the jar, and sniff or inhale. (Do this carefully at first to avoid irritating your nose and eyes.) Quickly replace the cap to keep the remaining aromatic substances from escaping. This treatment requires fresh-ground horseradish; most likely, it will lose its potency after four or five days.

HORSEMINT: In the folk medicine of southern Appalachia, horsemint (Monarda punctata) is a traditional treatment for hay fever. Horsemint may be inhaled, or you can drink it as a simple tea. Horsemint is not readily available in stores today, but its antiallergic constituent is probably the essential oil thymol. Scientific studies have shown that thymol reduces swelling in the bronchial tract, relaxes the trachea, and acts as an anti-inflammatory and mild antibacterial. The kitchen spice thyme also contains large

The Hair of the Dog That Bit You

In *Herbal Medicine Past and Present* (Volume I), by John K. Crellin and Jane Philpott, a traditional Appalachian herbalist named Tommie Bass, of northern Georgia, says: "You can make a tea from ragweed, or anything else you are allergic to, and drink 2 to 3 cupfuls while you have an allergy." According to Bass, who participated in a major study of folk medicine in the northern Georgia region during the 1980s, the method often works just "like an allergy shot."

Other folk remedies, originating in both Texas and the Ozark mountains, also call for the ingestion of substances to which you are allergic, such as locally grown bee pollen or honey. If you treat allergies in this manner, you may be taking a gamble, however. While the method undoubtedly works for some individuals, others may experience a worsening of allergies. And though rare, a life-threatening allergic reaction called anaphylaxis can occur from consuming pollen or teas from plants you are allergic to.

amounts of this aromatic oil and can be substituted for horsemint.

☞ DIRECTIONS: Place ½ ounce of ground thyme in a 1-pint jar and cover with boiling water. Close the jar tightly and let the mixture cool for half an hour. Remove the lid and inhale, taking a few deep breaths. Do this as needed throughout the day to help ease hay fever.

CHAMOMILE AND THYME OIL: German immigrants inhaled the fumes of chamomile tea (*Matricaria recutita*) to treat bouts of hay fever. In contemporary German naturopathic medicine, 3 to 5 drops of the essential oil of thyme is added to chamomile tea for the same purpose. (The action of thyme oil is described under the remedy

Horsemint, page 21.)
Chamomile contains the essential oil azulene and related oils that are anti-inflammatory and antiallergic, as well as the oil alpha-bisabolol, which is also an anti-inflammatory.

☞ DIRECTIONS: Place ½ ounce of chamomile flowers in a 1-quart jar. Fill two thirds of the jar with boiling water. Add 3 to 5 drops of essential oil of thyme. Cover and let cool for half an hour. Open the lid and inhale the fumes, taking a few deep breaths. Repeat as desired throughout the day. (Be careful of inhaling chamomile flower dust, because the pollen causes allergy in some people.)

MINT TEAS: Inhaling, drinking, or washing affected skin areas with mint teas can be accredited in this country to the folk medicine of the Seneca Indians. The plants used to make the teas are peppermint (Mentha piperita) and spearmint (Mentha spicata). In China, cornmint (Mentha arvensis),

which is similar in its chemical composition to peppermint, is used. (Mint teas have been used to treat allergies in China at least since the 7th century A.D.)

When consumed as a tea or inhaled, the essential oils in the mints act as a decongestant. When applied to the skin, the menthol in peppermint and cornmint produces a cooling sensation and reduces itching. (Spearmint contains little menthol, however, so it does not have this effect on the skin.) All three of the mints contain other anti-inflammatory and mild antibacterial constituents.

☞ DIRECTIONS: Place ½ ounce of dried mint leaves in a 1-quart jar. Fill two thirds of the jar with boiling water and cover the jar tightly. Let cool for half an hour. Strain and drink. The tea's fumes will also help relieve congestion.

EYEBRIGHT: The use of eyebright (Euphrasia officinalis) to treat allergies in the eastern United

States dates back at least 150 years and may have had its roots among German immigrants. At the turn of the century, Eclectic physicians, a group of M.D.s who used mostly herbs as medicines, also used eyebright to treat allergy symptoms among their patients (see sidebar, "Eclectic Medicine," page 25). During the same period, the pharmaceutical companies Parke Davis and Eli Lilly sold eyebright allergy preparations to the public. Eyebright is used today in Appalachia as a folk remedy for allergies.

Eyebright contains the constituents caffeic acid and ferulic acid, both of which have an anti-inflammatory effect. The caffeic acid also has specific antihistamine effects.

☞ DIRECTIONS: You can purchase eyebright tincture in a health food store or herb shop. Take a dropperful every three to four hours during the height of allergy season.

Another option is to make your own tincture. Place 2 ounces of dried eyebright leaves in a 1-pint jar and fill the jar with grain alcohol or 100 proof gin or vodka. Cover the jar and let it stand in a cool, dark place for three weeks, shaking the jar each day. After three weeks, strain and store the solution in the refrigerator. Take as directed above.

Bringing out Hives

In traditional African-American folk medicine, hives in a young baby are considered a good sign. It is believed that through hives, impurities in the body are released. In fact, some individuals believe that a fussy baby's mood can only improve if hives break out. Thus, catnip tea is sometimes given to relax a fussy baby and to help "bring out hives." Using catnip for this purpose is also a widespread practice among southern Appalachian whites, although it lacks any scientific verification.

Eclectic Medicine

The Eclectic movement was formed in the late 1820s and 1830s by medical doctors who were disgruntled with the medical methods used at the time, such as bloodletting and the administration of poisonous minerals like mercury. They sought knowledge of the "new" North American plants, ("new" compared to their knowledge of European plants) and turned to American Indian traditions and the folk medicine of the early states for inspiration. They formally named themselves "Eclectics" in the 1840s and began to experiment clinically with many herbal medicines. By 1900, the Eclectics had a number of medical schools throughout the country and produced sophisticated textbooks on clinical herbalism. During the first two decades of the 20th century, under pressure from the political organizations of more conventional doctors, the Eclectic schools lost their accreditation, and their graduates were denied licensing. The Eclectic Institute, the last Eclectic medical school, graduated the last group of Eclectic physicians in 1939.

HIVES AND ALLERGIC REACTIONS

BASIL TEA: A traditional Chinese folk remedy for treating hives is to bathe the skin in basil tea. Basil contains high amounts of caffeic acid, one of the key antiallergic constituents also contained in eyebright.

☞ DIRECTIONS: Place 1 ounce of dried basil leaves in a 1-quart jar and fill the jar with boiling water. Cover the jar tightly and let cool to room temperature. Use the solution as a wash for hives or itchy allergic skin rashes as often as needed.

ASAFOETIDA: Asafoetida (*Ferula assafoetida*), a relative of onions and garlic that is sometimes called "devil's dung," is a popular

Alabama folk remedy for hives. Asafoetida contains the volatile constituents ferulic acid and umbellifer-one, both of which have an anti-inflammatory effect. Umbelliferone also has an antiallergic effect.

☞ DIRECTIONS: Add ¼ teaspoon of asafoetida powder (available in many supermarkets in the spice section) to 4 tablespoons of warm castor oil. Mix well. Apply the solution directly to hives. Be aware that this material has a strong, garlic-like odor.

BAKING SODA BATHS: Taking a baking soda bath is an old New England folk remedy for soothing hives.

☞ DIRECTIONS: Place a few handfuls of baking soda in warm bath water and soak for twenty to thirty minutes. You can enjoy baking soda baths as often as you like.

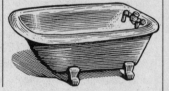

❧ Anxiety and ❧ Nervousness

▨ ▨ ▨

Everyone experiences some anxiety. Anxiety helps us stay alert and adapt to the ever-changing demands of our environment. Anxiety is really the body's "early warning system" against harm. When we feel danger, the alarm goes off to warn us and prevent injury. The body responds immediately to the alarm emotionally, physically, and behaviorally. Emotionally, we may feel fear, doom, or anger. Physically, our hearts race, muscles tense, breathing becomes rapid, and palms and feet start to sweat. We respond behaviorally by getting ready to fight or flee from danger.

The anxiety warning system works fine when there's clear and present danger, but anxiety can become a problem for people when they perceive harmless situations or people as threatening.

There is no single reason why some people experience episodes of chronic anxiety. Some of these individuals will benefit from visiting a psychotherapist, who can help them sort out internal conflicts or past conditioning that may be causing the emotional state. Any physical change, such as illness, can also cause anxiety. Anemia, diabetes, premenstrual syndrome, menopause, thyroid disorder, hypoglycemia, pulmonary disease, endocrine tumors, and other conditions can cause anxiety symptoms. Other individuals simply

need to improve their nutrition and lifestyle—anxiety can be the symptom of several nutrient deficiencies or lifestyle habits that are common in modern society.

One of the most commonly overlooked causes of anxiety and nervousness in modern life is related to caffeine consumption. Even moderate amounts of caffeine can create nervous symptoms severe enough to earn a diagnosis of chronic anxiety—and a subsequent prescription of sedative drugs or referral to a therapist.

One scientific theory suggests that anxiety is closely associated with the balance of the substances lactate and pyruvate in the body. These two substances are associated with energy production within the cells, and high lactate levels may cause anxiety. Alcohol, caffeine, and sugar all increase lactate levels, and the B-vitamins niacin and thiamine and the mineral magnesium all lower it. Deficiencies of the B-vitamins as well as omega-

3 fatty acids, such as occur naturally in fish and wild game, may thus contribute to anxiety.

Conventional treatment of anxiety is primarily with drugs of the benzodiazepine class, such as Valium and Xanax. Anxiety patients are often treated by psychotherapists as well. Below are some natural remedies you can try to help ease feelings of stress and anxiety.

Remedies

VALERIAN: In folk medicine, valerian is considered a universal sedative. The Greeks used valerian as a relaxant and antispasmodic. The herb was also used in the folk medicine of India, Tibet, and Japan. Today, Mexicans and Mexican-Americans use varieties of the plant native to their regions. An African-American folk remedy from Louisiana is to put valerian root in a pillow and inhale its fragrance as you sleep. Valerian continues to be used as a sedative among today's Appalachians as well.

Valeriana officinalis, the European variety of the plant, was brought to the eastern colonies by immigrants for cultivation. It has subsequently become native in the eastern United States. Valerian is recognized today as an official medicine for nervousness and anxiety by the German government. Its suspected active constituents are its essential oils. Valerian has proven to be as effective as the sedative Valium

Driving Out Evil Spirits

Several of the sedative herbs in this section have been used traditionally to "drive out evil spirits" or to treat epilepsy, which in ancient times was considered to be a form of possession. Both valerian and rosemary are still used today in ritual purifications in southwestern and Mexican folk medicine.

in some clinical trials, although it has no relationship chemically to that drug.

☞ DIRECTIONS: Place 2 to 3 teaspoons of dried chopped valerian root in a cup and cover with boiling water. Cover the cup and let stand for fifteen minutes. Drink 2 to 3 cups a day for up to three weeks. Individuals who use valerian for longer than three weeks, or who use valerian to help them get to sleep, can ultimately develop lethargy and experience hangover-like effects.

Here is a recipe from gypsy folk medicine for valerian wine: Take 2 handfuls of chopped valerian root, 1 whole clove, 1 orange rind, 1 sprig of rosemary, and 1 quart of dry white wine. Place the dried herbs in a 1-quart jar and cover with the wine. Seal the container and allow to stand in a cool dark place for one cycle of the moon. Strain and store. Take 1 tablespoon of the mixture three times a day for up to three weeks. It should be noted that valerian has a very disagreeable odor.

VALERIAN AND HOP: German immigrants of the late 18th century treated nervousness with a mixture of equal portions of valerian (*Valeriana officinalis*) and hop (*Humulus lupulus*). Commercial combinations of these two herbs are still popular in Germany today. Hop has also been used as a sedative among British immigrants, Seventh Day Adventists, Indiana farmers, and residents of the American Southwest.

☞ DIRECTIONS: Mix equal amounts by volume of dried and chopped valerian root and hop in a bowl. Place 1 tablespoon of the mixture in a cup and fill the cup with boiling water. Cover the cup and let stand for twenty minutes. Strain and drink 3 cups a day. Take nightly for up to three weeks.

CATNIP: Catnip tea has been used as a popular sleep aid in America since *continued on page 32*

Birth Order and Healing Powers

▨ ▨ ▨

In the modern world, special abilities are attributed to those who have received specialized training. Physicians, with their many years of schooling, are a good example of these experts. Although healing has always involved learning, it has not always been a matter of mastering facts and technique. Folk healers, for example, differ from medical doctors in that they believe they have been led to their work by a Divine call. For that reason, the power given to folk healers has often been considered by the community as far more important than what they have actually studied or done.

For many healers, their calling is indicated by their circumstances of birth. Probably the best known birth indication of healing power is being the "seventh son of a seventh son." Women are healers in folk tradition, too, and seventh daughters are seen as having power also. Among Gypsies, seventh daughters are said to be especially talented fortune-tellers. Abilities often ascribed to seventh children include stopping blood flow, curing whooping cough, and curing thrush, which is a yeast infection of the mouth that was sometimes quite serious in infants before modern treatment was readily available.

These were common medical emergencies, and respect for the healing abilities of seventh children was great. The powers of these children were not limited to healing, however, even though seventh sons were often nicknamed "Doc." Their talents could also be related to music. An example is Doc Watson, a gifted folk guitarist and singer, now quite famous, named for his birth order. In French tradition, a seventh child is said to have "the gift of the lily," which includes a kind of clairvoyance or second sight.

Being born after the death of one's father—sometimes called a "post-humous child"—was another circumstance of birth said to give healing power. In Illinois, folk tradition attributes the same healing powers to both post-humous children and those children who have never seen their father for other reasons. In Georgia, a belief has been recorded that connects the post-humous child with the power of seven, stating that "sore mouth among children," possibly a reference to thrush, can be cured by seven sips of water from the shoe of one who was born after her or his father died.

> For many healers, their calling is indicated by their circumstances of birth. Probably the best birth indication of healing power is being the "seventh son of a seventh son."

The most dramatic birth circumstance to convey healing power is being born with a "caul," or "veil." A caul is a portion of the amnion, the membrane that covers the fetus in the womb. Since ancient times, among both Romans and Jews, a baby born with this membrane adhering to its head has been believed to have special powers. It was also believed that the caul itself had supernatural powers and protected whoever owned it from demons. This belief made the caul a valuable commodity—one that was bought and sold up through the 19th century.

the arrival of European immigrants in New England. The popularity of the tea spread rapidly in the New World, and American Indians soon adopted its use. The Onondaga and Cayuga Indian tribes used catnip to calm restless children, and European New Englanders gave it to adults for nervous disorders, including nervous breakdown. Today, catnip remains a common folk remedy among residents of Appalachia.

☞ DIRECTIONS: Place 1 to 3 teaspoons of the dried herb in a cup and cover with boiling water. Cover the cup and let stand for ten minutes. Strain and drink 3 cups a day. Use as needed.

CELERY AND ONIONS: Some contemporary Indiana residents, according to a survey of folk remedies in the state, suggested eating celery and onions

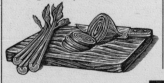

to overcome nervousness. Both celery and onions contain large amounts of potassium and folic acid. Studies have shown that deficiencies of each of these nutrients can cause fatigue, insomnia, and nervousness.

☞ DIRECTIONS: Eat 2 cups of either celery or onions, or a combination of the two, raw or cooked, with each meal for a week.

SKULLCAP: More than a hundred species of skullcap (Scutellaria spp.) grow throughout the world. North American varieties of the herb were used by American Indian tribes such as the Penobscot, Iroquois, and Cherokee to treat diarrhea and heart disease and to promote menstruation and eliminate afterbirth. Skullcap received its common name, mad dog weed, in the 18th century, when the herb was widely prescribed as a cure for rabies. Skullcap is still used today in Appalachian folk medicine as a sedative. The suspected medicinal constituents are flavonoids and an essential oil.

☞ DIRECTIONS: Put 2 or 3 teaspoonfuls of dried skullcap leaves in a cup and fill with boiling water. Cover and let steep for fifteen minutes. Strain and drink 3 to 4 cups a day as needed.

ROSEMARY: European and Spanish immigrants brought the herb rosemary (*Rosmarinus officinalis*) with them to cultivate in the New World. Rosemary was later used by early Californians to rid the body of "evil spirits" or to treat epilepsy, which in ancient times was considered to be a form of possession.

Rosemary has long been used in European and Chinese folk medicine to calm the nerves. Medical experts in the United States continue to recommend rosemary to treat nervous conditions. Rosemary's analgesic and antispasmodic properties are also recognized by the German government; the herb is used there as an official medical treatment for spastic conditions, including epilepsy.

☞ DIRECTIONS: Add 1 or 2 teaspoons of the dried herb to a cup and fill the cup with boiling water. Cover the cup and let stand ten minutes. Strain and drink 2 to 3 cups a day as needed.

PASSION FLOWER: Of 19 passion flower species worldwide, eight have been used as sedatives by various cultures. Passion flower (*Passiflora incarnata*) is native from Florida to Texas and may also be found as far north as Missouri. The herb is abundant in South America; it's long-time use as a sedative there is recorded in Brazilian folk medicine.

The passion flower species *P. incarnata* was introduced into American professional medicine in 1840 after medical doctors in Mississippi experimented with it and demonstrated its sedative effects. Thereafter the herb was mainly used by doctors of the Eclectic school (see

American Ginseng

American ginseng (*Panax quinquefolius*) grows in the Appalachian Mountains and has long been used as a sedative and tonic by the people who live there. A related species of ginseng, Panax ginseng, is perhaps the most famous tonic herb in China, although Chinese herbalists use that plant as a stimulant rather than a sedative.

In the early 1700s, Jesuit priests noticed American ginseng growing in the Canadian woods and initiated export of the plant to China. Some 100,000 tons have been shipped there in the last 250 years. Ginseng harvesting and export became an important economic force in the early American colonies, among American Indians and traders alike. Wild ginseng is now almost extinct in North America, but large quantities are grown commercially in Michigan and Wisconsin, mostly for export to China, where demand for it remains high.

"Eclectic Medicine," page 25). Passion flower is still popularly used as a sedative among residents of southern Appalachia and among the Amish. The herb is also widely cultivated in Europe for medicinal purposes; it has been approved by the German government as a sedative medicine.

Passion flower is a gentle sedative and is often combined with other plants. Most likely, its active constituent is an alkaloid, called passiflorine (or harmane).

☞ DIRECTIONS: Place 1 heaping teaspoon of dried passion flower in a cup, fill the cup with boiling water, cover, and steep ten minutes. Strain and drink as needed.

MOTHERWORT: Motherwort is a mild relaxing agent often recommended by herbalists to reduce anxiety and depression and treat nervousness, insomnia, heart palpitations, and rapid heart rate. Motherwort (*Leonurus cardiaca*) has been used in Europe since antiquity as a sedative and to treat menstrual irregularities. Motherwort probably came to North America with physicians among the British colonists. American Indian tribes later adopted the herb's medicinal uses.

Today, in Germany, motherwort is an approved medicine for treating anxiety. It is also used in contemporary Chinese medicine for the same purpose. The herb contains a chemical called leonurine, which may encourage uterine contractions, however. Thus, you will want to avoid motherwort if you are pregnant or trying to conceive.

☞ DIRECTIONS: Place 1 to 2 teaspoons of motherwort herb in a cup and fill the cup with boiling water. Cover the cup and let stand for ten to fifteen minutes. Strain and drink. The tea's taste is bitter, so you may wish to mix it with other herbs. Don't drink more than 2 to 3 cups a day.

❦ Arthritis ❧

▦ ▦ ▦

In a nutshell, arthritis means "inflammation of the joints." Rheumatism is an old medical term that was used to describe inflammation of either joints or muscles. Rheum was thought to be a watery mucus-like secretion, sometimes brought on by cold weather. Joint or muscle pain was thought to be caused by such secretions trapped in the tissues. Although the concept is not far from the truth—inflammation is usually accompanied by swelling and a build-up of fluid—the modern explanation of arthritis is much more precise.

Today's medical experts suggest there are at least 23 varieties of arthritis, including rheumatoid arthritis and osteoarthritis, the two most common types. With osteoarthritis—sometimes called degener-ative joint disease, or DJD—there is a gradual wearing away of cartilage in the joints. Healthy cartilage is the elastic tissue that lines and cushions the joints and allows bones to move smoothly against one another. When this cartilage deteriorates, the bones rub together, causing pain and swelling. Permanent damage and stiffness of the joints is possible.

Aspirin-like Compounds in Plants

Over the past hundred years, aspirin has been one of the most common treatments for inflammatory arthritis. Today we have a wide variety of aspirin-like drugs, such as ibuprofen and naproxen, which are collectively called non-steroidal anti-inflammatory drugs, or NSAIDs.

Aspirin was developed as a less toxic substitute for methyl-salicylate, which comes from the wintergreen plant (*Gaulteria procumbens*). Wintergreen was used as a traditional American Indian treatment for rheumatism and headache. Aspirin-like compounds are also contained in the herbs black cohosh (*Cimicifuga racemosa*), black haw (*Viburnum prunifolium*), pipsissewa (*Chimaphila umbellata*), and white willow bark (*Salix alba*). Therapeutically, these herbs are not as powerful as aspirin or today's NSAIDs, but they are less likely to cause gastrointestinal bleeding, a side effect that afflicts from two to four percent of regular NSAID users and causes 2,000 to 3,000 deaths a year.

Rheumatoid arthritis can attack at any age. This form of arthritis affects all the connective tissues, as well as other organs. The precise cause of rheumatoid arthritis is unknown. Some researchers believe that a virus triggers the disease, causing an autoimmune response whereby the body attacks its own tissues. However, evidence for this theory is inconclusive. What is confirmed is the progression of the condition. First, the synovium (the thin membrane that lines and lubricates the joint) becomes inflamed. The inflammation eventually destroys the cartilage. As scar tissue gradually replaces the damaged cartilage, the joint becomes misshaped and rigid. Rheumatoid arthritis may damage the heart, lungs, nerves, and eyes.

A medical examination and diagnosis is required to identify the cause and nature of any chronic joint or muscular pain. Other "rheumatic" diseases include arthralgia (pain in a joint), fibrositis ("muscular rheumatism"), and synovitis (inflammation of the joint membrane).

There is no simple cure for arthritis. Conventional treatment for chronic joint pain is to use drugs to suppress the inflammation in order to reduce pain and also prevent tissue destruction. Usually, simple aspirin-related pain medications, called nonsteroidal anti-inflammatory drugs (NSAIDs), are first prescribed. Corticosteroids may be prescribed for more serious illness, especially when tissue destruction is evident. In about 15 percent of rheumatoid arthritis cases, these measures are ineffective, and stronger substances are used. Oral or injectable gold may prove helpful in treating rheumatoid arthritis. Some drugs usually used for cancer treatment may also be helpful.

Alternative physicians usually treat arthritis by recommending short fasts, screening for food allergies, recommending avoidance of processed foods, introducing fish and fish oils to the diet as well as anti-inflammatory herbal and nutritional supplements, and using natural methods to improve digestion. Alternative physicians may also recommend the substance glucosamine sulfate, which provides natural building blocks for cartilage, as a dietary supplement for those suffering from osteoarthritis. Scientific studies have suggested that supplementation with B vitamins, vitamin E, and some multiminerals (including the trace elements copper and selenium) may also improve the disease. On the other hand, studies have shown that nightshade vegetables—potatoes, tomatoes, bell peppers, and chili peppers—may provoke joint pain.

Very few of the herbs or foods recommended in folk literature for treating arthritis have been tested clinically for anti-inflammatory effects. Many of these herbs and foods contain plant constituents for which such anti-inflammatory effects are known, however.

Remedies

CELERY: The remedy of eating raw or cooked celery seeds (*Apium graveolens*) or large amounts of the celery plant to treat rheumatism arrived in North America with the British and German immigrants. Using celery to treat rheumatism persists today in North American professional herbalism. Various parts of the celery plant contain more than 25 different anti-inflammatory compounds. And, taken as a food, celery is rich in minerals: A cup of celery contains more than 340 milligrams of potassium. (A potassium deficiency may contribute to some symptoms of arthritis.)

Potato Magic

A magical arthritis remedy from the Appalachians, and also from rural Louisiana, is to carry a potato around with you. In fact, some say, in order for the remedy to work, the potato must be carried in the right-hand pants pocket; others insist that you must carry an Irish potato.

☞ DIRECTIONS: Place 1 teaspoon of celery seeds in a cup. Fill the cup with boiling water. Cover and let stand for fifteen minutes. Strain and drink. Drink 3 cups a day during an acute arthritis attack.

ANGELICA: Angelica (*Angelica archangelica*), an herb that has been used in European folk medicine since antiquity, can be used to treat arthritis. The Western variety of angelica has 12 anti-inflammatory constituents, ten antispasmodic (muscle relaxant) constituents, and five anodyne (pain-relieving) ones. The Chinese sometimes use their native variety of the plant (*Angelica sinensis*) for the same purpose. The Chinese species is sold in North America under the names *dang gui* or *dong quai*.

☞ DIRECTIONS: Place 1 tablespoon of the cut roots of either species of angelica in 1 pint of water and bring to a boil. Cover and boil for two minutes. Remove from heat and let stand, covered, until the water cools to room temperature. Strain and drink the tea in 3 doses during the day for two to three weeks at a time. Then, take a break for seven to ten days and start the treatment again if desired.

ROSEMARY: A collection of remedies by folklorist Clarence Meyer called *American Folk Medicine* suggests drinking rosemary tea to treat arthritis. The same remedy is used in the contemporary folk medicine of the Coahuila Indians in Mexico. Rosemary has not been tested

Counterirritants and Arthritis

A universal approach to relieving arthritis pain in all cultures is the application of a counterirritant, or substance that irritates and inflames the skin over the painful area. Cayenne pepper, pine pitch, bee and scorpion stings, and modern over-the-counter remedies such as Ben Gay ointment are all used for this purpose. Physiological tests show that such treatments increase blood flow to the area by as much as four times and also increase blood flow and temperature in the muscles beneath the skin.

Any relief from such treatments is due to this increase of circulation to the area. Counterirritation may also increase local or systemic levels of endorphins, natural pain-killing substances that can be more potent than opiates.

in clinical trials, but it was used to relieve pain and spasm by doctors of the Physiomedicalist school, a group of M.D.s in the second half of the 19th century who used only herbs when treating patients. The plant's leaves contain four anti-inflammatory substances— carnosol, oleanolic acid, rosmarinic acid, and ursolic acid. Carnosol acts on the same anti-inflammatory pathways as both steroids and aspirin, oleanolic acid has been marketed as an antioxidant in China, rosmarinic acid acts as an anti-inflammatory, and ursolic acid, which makes up about four percent of the plant by weight, has been shown to have antiarthritic effects in animal trials.

☞ DIRECTIONS: Put ½ ounce of rosemary leaves in a 1-quart canning jar and fill the jar with boiling water. Cover tightly and let stand for thirty minutes. Drink a cup of the hot tea before going to bed and have another cupful in the morning before breakfast. Do this for two to three weeks, and then take a break for seven to ten days before starting the treatment again.

WINTERGREEN: Wintergreen *(Gaulteria procumbens)* was used to treat arthritis by the Delaware, Menominee, Ojibwa, Potawatomi, and Iroquois Indian tribes. The plant was accepted in the United States as an official medicine for arthritis in 1820; it is still included—in the form of wintergreen oil—in the *United States Pharmacopoeia* today. The chief active pain-relieving constituent in wintergreen is methyl-salicylate. This compound can be toxic when consumed in concentrated wintergreen oil, even when applied to the skin, so, if you want to use this plant, stick with using the dried herb. (Aspirin was developed as a safer alternative to methyl-salicylate.)
    ☞ DIRECTIONS: Place 1 or 2 teaspoons of dried wintergreen leaves in a

cup and cover with boiling water. Cover the cup and let steep for fifteen minutes. Strain and drink 3 cups a day. Do this for two to three weeks, and then take a break for seven to ten days before starting again.

BLACK COHOSH: An American Indian treatment for arthritis, in both the Seneca and Cherokee tribes, involved using the root of black cohosh *(Cimicifuga racemosa)*. White settlers in the eastern states eventually adopted the plant's use, as did the Eclectic physicians of the last century (see sidebar, "Eclectic Medicine," page 25). There are five species in the *Cimicifuga* genus worldwide that have been used to treat rheumatism. Black cohosh contains aspirin-like substances as well as other anti-inflammatory and antispasmodic constituents.
    ☞ DIRECTIONS: Simmer 1 teaspoon of black cohosh root in 1 cup of boiling water for twenty

minutes. Strain and drink the tea in 2 divided doses during the day. Do this for two to three weeks, and then take a break for seven to ten days before starting the treatment again.

HOP TEA: Hop is native to Europe and can be found in vacant fields and along rivers there. The Pilgrims brought hop (*Humulus lupulus*) to Massachusetts, and it quickly spread south to Virginia. The hop plant contains at least 22 constituents that have anti-inflammatory activities, including several that act through the same cellular mechanisms as steroid drugs. Four constituents have antispasmodic properties, and ten may act as sedatives. The fresher the plant, the

better. Today, a popular remedy for rheumatism in Mexico and the American Southwest is hop tea.

☞ DIRECTIONS: Place 2 or 3 teaspoons of hop leaves in a cup and fill with boiling water. Cover the cup and let stand for fifteen minutes. Drink the tea while it's warm. The tea is bitter. Drink 1 to 3 cups between dinner and bedtime as needed.

ALFALFA: Alfalfa (*Medicago sativa*) is often promoted in health food stores as an arthritis remedy—in the form of capsulated alfalfa powder. Alfalfa contains l-canavanine, however, an amino acid that can cause symptoms that are similar to those of systemic lupus, an autoimmune disease that can also cause joint pain. Some scientific studies show that these symptoms can occur in both animals and humans as a result of eating alfalfa. Thus, the remedy below is best taken in the form of a tea rather than powder; the amino

Blood Purifiers

Traditional "blood purifiers" mentioned in Appalachian folk literature as being treatments for arthritis include sassafras (*Sassafras albidum*), sarsaparilla (*Smilax officinalis*), and burdock (*Arctium lappa, Arctium minus*). Residents in the American Southwest insist red clover (*Trifolium pratense*) and yerba mansa (*Anemopsis californicum*) do the trick. Practitioners of folk medicine in New York recommend dandelion root (*Taraxacum officinale*) as the best treatment for arthritis.

acid is not present to any significant amount in alfalfa tea. Alfalfa tea is rich with nutritive minerals. It is a recommended folk remedy for arthritis in southern Appalachia.

☞ DIRECTIONS: Place 1 ounce of alfalfa tea in a pot. Cover with 1 quart of water and boil for thirty minutes. Strain and drink the quart throughout the day. Do this for two to three weeks, and then take a break for seven to ten days before starting again.

PINE PITCH AND TURPENTINE: American Indians of the Six Nations tribes of the northeastern United States and southeastern Canada used pine pitch (congealed pine sap) applied externally as a counterirritant treatment for arthritis (see sidebar, "Counterirritants and Arthritis," page 40). The practice was later adopted by residents of Appalachia. Today, turpentine, which is made from pine pitch, is used there for the same purpose.

☞ DIRECTIONS: Mix a small amount of turpentine with lard or vegetable oil to keep it from burning the skin. Apply over the area of the arthritis pain. Leave it on for ten to twenty minutes. Wipe off.

MUSTARD PLASTER: Perhaps the most famous of the counterirritant treatments for arthritis is the mustard plaster. This treatment is used throughout Europe and also in Appalachia and China. The irritating substance in mustard is allyl-isothyocyanate, which is related to the acrid substances in garlic and onions. This constituent is not activated, however, until the seeds are crushed and mixed with some liquid. Only then does the mustard produce the irritation necessary for the counterirritant effect.

☞ DIRECTIONS: Crush the seeds of white or brown mustard *(Brassica alba, Brassica juncea)* or grind them in a seed grinder. Moisten the mixture with vinegar, then sprinkle with flour. Spread the mixture on a cloth. Place the cloth, poultice side down, on the skin. Leave on for no more than twenty minutes.

Chaparral

Chaparral (*Larrea tridentata*) is widely promoted in health food stores as a treatment for arthritis. In the early 1990s, reports of liver toxicity for chaparral appeared in scientific documents, and 18 cases of adverse effects to chaparral have since been reported to the Food and Drug Administration (FDA). Two of those patients required liver transplants. The individuals who were poisoned took powdered chaparral in the form of capsules, ingesting toxic constituents that are not present in the traditional teas.

Chaparral was widely used by the American Indians of the Southwest. These Indian groups used chaparral either externally as a wash or internally as a tea, however; they did not take it in the form of powdered capsules. Pima Indians recommended using only the new growing green parts of the plant for the tea, a consideration not always followed in today's herb commerce where old dire leaves are just as likely to be used.

Remove if the poultice becomes uncomfortable. After removing the poultice, wash the affected area.

HOT PEPPERS: Cayenne pepper *(Capsicum spp.)* appears in counterirritant potions in China, the American Southwest, and throughout Ohio, Indiana, and Illinois. External and internal use of cayenne pepper was a key element of Thomsonian herbalism, which was popular throughout rural New England and the Midwest in the early 1800s. Cayenne works by reducing substance P, a chemical that carries pain messages from the skin's nerve endings, so it reduces pain when applied topically. Try this simple cayenne liniment.

☞ DIRECTIONS: Place 1 ounce of cayenne pepper in 1 quart of rubbing alcohol (a poison not for internal use). Let stand for three weeks, shaking the bottle each day. Then, using a cloth, apply to the affected area during acute attacks of pain. Leave the solution in place for ten to twenty minutes, then wipe clean.

GINSENG LIQUOR: The Iroquois Indians used American ginseng *(Panax quinquefolius)* as a treatment for rheumatism. Today, the Chinese use the herb for the same purpose. Be sure to use American ginseng, however, not Asian ginseng *(Panax ginseng);* Asian ginseng can actually aggravate the pain of arthritis. Ginseng contains constituents called ginsenosides, which have a variety of pharmacological actions. Both the American and Asian varieties of the plant are classified as adaptogens, meaning that they increase the body's ability to handle a wide variety of stresses. The Iroquois Indians made a tea of the plant's roots and added whiskey. You might prefer the Chinese formula below.

☞ DIRECTIONS: Chop 3½ ounces of ginseng and place in 1 quart of liquor
continued on page 50

Wild Animal Magic

While folk medicine uses domestic animals for both natural and magical purposes, wild animals are almost always used for magical reasons. This may be because many wild animals are more difficult to obtain. This seems especially likely because those wild animals that are easily accessible, especially insects and spiders, have more often been put to natural uses.

BIRDS: Birds' nests, which are relatively easy to find, have been linked magically with headache. Folklorists in several different parts of the United States have discovered the belief that if discarded human hair is used by birds to build a nest, its former owner will get a headache. The reverse effect—and opposite logic—is also found. It is believed by some that headaches can be prevented by placing your first pulled tooth in a bird's nest.

MOLES: Of all the wild mammals used in folk medicine, the lowly mole has perhaps the longest and most peculiar history. Moles are small rodents that live underground and eat insects. In ancient times the mole was venerated from India to Europe as spiritually powerful. In Greece, the name of the god of healing, Asclepias, is derived from the ancient Greek word for mole. This veneration is in part due to the mole's ability to live so completely underground—which is unique

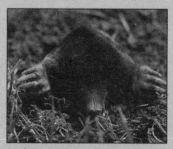

In folk medicine, the mole is used to cure.

among mammals—and the fact that the powers of fertility and mystery have been attributed to the underground world. For these reasons, the mole occupies a special place in occult folk medicine. One means of acquiring the power to heal is to hold a mole tightly in your hand and suffocate it. Some people believe that, as the mole dies, its power is transferred to the one who holds it. This belief can still be encountered in many rural parts of the United States. Most remedies that use moles involve injury or death to the animal. A tooth extracted from a live mole and worn around the neck is said to prevent toothache (a belief also common in ancient Greece and Rome). A mole's foot worn around the neck as an amulet is supposed to prevent the pain of teething. In North Car-

Mysterious Little Creatures

Although we may not think of them in this way, earthworms are a kind of wild animal. And they are readily available—as anyone who has ever collected fishing bait or dug up a garden plot knows. Earthworms are mysterious little creatures, which is a plus in folk medicine. Although most people today may find the idea disgusting, a common topical remedy was once made by cooking earthworms in a skillet and saving the oil. No more appetizing is this remedy for quinsy (severe tonsillitis), which was reported in the 1930s in Pennsylvania: Fill a flannel cloth with live earthworms and pin it around the patient's neck. The worms will draw out the soreness and die. Earthworms are also said to die when they come in contact with the left side of a seventh son of a seventh son, an indication of the great power bestowed by this birth order.

olina, the string holding the mole paw must be black, and, in some cases, the paw is supposed to be bitten off a live mole. The use of "moleskin" to protect sore and blistered skin is the one connection that exists between moles and contemporary medicine. Fortunately the moleskin purchased in pharmacies today is a kind of cotton twill, not the result of animal sacrifice!

MUSKRATS: Another readily accessible wild animal is the muskrat, widely trapped for its fur. In Maryland, a fresh muskrat skin was used to prevent colds by sewing the bloody side of the skin to red flannel. The flannel side was then worn next to the skin until it fell off of its own accord. The effect was said to be enhanced by first rubbing the patient with goose grease.

TOADS: Toads, widely and mistakenly believed to cause warts, figure very prominently in traditional remedies. Many of these treatments seem to involve magical transfer of an illness to a toad or to a toad's body part. The following remedy for a foot wound that won't heal comes from Pennsylvania: Tie a linen thread around the foot of a toad, cut off the foot, and tie it to your sore leg. Leave the thread in place until it falls off, and the wound will be healed. In Georgia, local legend has it that whooping cough can be cured by tying a toad to the patient's bedpost. And in the folk medicine of California, asthma is thought to be cured by having the patient spit into a toad's mouth. In North Carolina, some think malaria can be relieved by blowing into a toad's mouth. Finally,

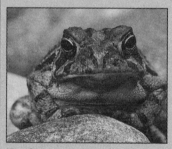

Toads are used to remedy various illnesses.

in Utah, it is said that toads can suck cancer right out of the body.

SNAKES: Snakes, and the oil rendered from them, have long been prominent in American folk medicine. So much so that the term "snake oil" is synonymous with fraudulent and useless remedies. This is due to the practices of quacks and medicine peddlers in the late 19th century. Snakes and snake oil, however, have also been important in authentic folk traditions. According to some African-American traditions, snake bones can be used as an amulet to cure toothache. In Colorado, it is said that if a person with a goiter wears a snake around his neck, the snake will take the goiter when it crawls away. (The exact type of snake was not specified but, presumably, it would have to be of the nonpoisonous variety.)

After snake oil, snakeskin is the most widely used part of the snake in folk remedies. In Maryland, it is said that snakeskin worn around the foot will ease cramps. Snakeskin has been worn in many parts of the country to alleviate rheumatism. And one odd medicinal function for snakes reported from southern Illinois says that rheumatism can be frightened out of a patient either by a tornado or by a water moccasin snake!

EELS: Even though fishing has been popular for food and sport through the centuries, fish remedies are relatively scarce in folk medicine. Those folk remedies that do involve fish often focus on eels. The Pennsylvania Germans say alcoholism can be cured by drinking whisky through which a live eel has passed. The Pennsylvania Germans also tie an eel skin around the arm to remedy a nosebleed. The most common use of eel skin is for treating joint pain, however. In Pennsylvania, it is believed that the skin of an eel, especially one caught in March, will provide relief when applied to a sprain. In Georgia, eel skin is combined with the widely used copper bracelet to cure arthritis.

Diuretic Herbs

Taking diuretic herbs as a treatment for arthritis has been recommended in various customs throughout the world; in North America, it was prescribed by physicians of the last century. The European colonists introduced the use of celery seed (*Apium graveolens*) to the eastern colonies as a diuretic and antirheumatic. The Seneca Indians used horsetail (*Equisetum arvense*) as a diuretic to treat arthritis, the Aztec Indians of Mexico used corn silk (*Zea mays*), and the Allegheny tribe used parsley (*Petroselenium sativum*). The Seneca and Pacific Northwest Indian tribes recommended pipsissewa (*Chimaphila umbellata*). Various eastern Indian groups took cramp bark (*Viburnum opulus*) and black haw (*Viburnum prunifolium*).

The rationale for this diuretic prescription is not clear, but its use remains widespread. Contemporary Appalachians use pipsissewa as well as Joe-Pye weed (*Eupatorium purpureum*). Pipsissewa, cramp bark, and black haw, in addition to their diuretic properties, also contain aspirin-like anti-inflammatory compounds.

like vodka. Let the mixture stand for five to six weeks in a cool dark place, turning the container frequently. Strain and take 1 ounce of the liquid after dinner or before bedtime every night for up to three months. Then, take a break for two weeks before starting the treatment again.

COPPER BRACELETS: The recommendation for arthritis patients to wear copper bracelets is common throughout European and American folk literature. Copper is a nutrient that may play a role in modifying arthritis. The nutrient takes part in key antioxidant systems that help prevent inflammation and is also necessary for the formation of connective tissue. The normal daily requirement of copper for an adult is 1.5 to 3 milligrams, but that requirement may be higher in patients with rheumatoid arthritis (but not osteoarthritis). A 1976 clinical trial demonstrated that copper bracelets could be an effective treatment for arthritis. Patients in the trial who wore copper bracelets had fewer symptoms than those who wore colored aluminum look-alikes. The researchers also found that the bracelets lost as much as 1.7 milligrams of copper a day, some of which may have dissolved in the individual's sweat and been absorbed through the skin.

☞ DIRECTIONS: Wear a copper bracelet around your wrist or ankle—the more surface area the bracelet covers, the better. (It is unlikely to absorb too much copper. Copper toxicity occurs after ingesting about 60 milligrams of copper, an amount that is many times more than

Dog Nap

A widespread folk practice to cure rheumatism is to sleep with a dog, with the animal resting against the affected area. In Mexico and the American Southwest, the dog is sometimes shaved. Physiologically, this may be an alternative to a hot water bottle or a heating pad, because the heat from the dog's body keeps the area warm. The practice has a darker side, however. Some cultures believe that the disease will go into the dog, the patient will be cured, and the dog will die. This use and superstition is also recorded in the medical practices of some southern African Americans as well as in the folk medicine of residents of North Carolina, Kentucky, Indiana, Illinois, Texas, Kansas, and Nebraska.

what is found in copper jewelry.)

EPSOM SALTS: In the town of Epsom, England, in 1618, a substance called magnesium sulfate was found in abundance in spring water. The colonists brought the substance, named Epsom salts, to this country. Magnesium has both anti-inflammatory and anti-arthritic properties and it can be absorbed through the skin. Magnesium is one of the most important of the essential minerals in the body, and it is commonly deficient in the American diet. A New England remedy for arthritis is a hot bath of Epsom salts. The heat of the bath can increase circulation and reduce the swelling of arthritis.

☞ DIRECTIONS: Fill a bathtub with water as hot as you can stand. Add 2 cups of Epsom salts. Bathe for thirty minutes, adding hot water as necessary to keep the temperature warm. Do this daily as often as you'd like. (If you are pregnant or have cardiovascular disease, however, consult your doctor before taking very hot baths.)

HYDROTHERAPY: Water treatments for arthritis, which have become popular throughout the United States in the last century, invariably involve heat. Hot water or steam increases the circulation, which in turn can reduce local inflammation and swelling. These water techniques are used today in parts of Appalachia and among the Seventh Day Adventists.

☞ DIRECTIONS: Try one of the following treatments: Take a steam bath in a sauna. Soak in a hot tub, or, if there is one in your area, a hot spring. You can also try placing hot towels on the afflicted area.

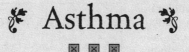

Asthma

Asthma now affects some fourteen million Americans and claims about five thousand lives a year. Asthma is the most common chronic disease among children, affecting one in five. Because it may be a life-threatening condition, any individual with asthma should be under the care of a physician. Asthma is a respiratory disorder marked by unpredictable periods of acute breathlessness and wheezing. Asthma attacks can last from less than an hour to a week or more and can strike frequently or only every few years. Attacks may be mild or severe and can occur at any time, even during sleep.

The difficult breathing occurs when the small respiratory tubes called bronchioles constrict or become clogged with mucus or when the membranes lining the bronchioles become swollen. When this happens, stale air cannot be fully exhaled but stays trapped in the lungs, so that less fresh air can be inhaled.

Asthma attacks can result from oversensitivity of the bronchial system to a variety of outside substances or conditions. About half of all asthma attacks are triggered by allergies to such substances as dust, smoke, pollen, feathers, pet hair, insects, mold spores, and a variety of foods and drugs. The allergic trigger cannot always be identified, and sometimes food allergens complicate the picture. An individual who is allergic to a specific food may experience "allergic overload" when consuming it and then overreact to a simple pollen or other airborne allergen that normally would not cause a serious problem. Attacks not related to allergies can be set off by strenuous exercise, breathing cold air, stress, and infections of the respiratory tract.

Modern physicians treat asthma with drugs delivered by inhalers, including, in serious cases, steroid drugs. Recent research has demonstrated that prolonged use of inhaled steroids can cause severe side effects similar to those experienced by users of oral steroids, however. Inhaled steroids nevertheless remain an essential and sometimes lifesaving part of treatment for severe asthma.

Why does the body overreact to a simple allergen? One possible explanation is a deficiency of the body's natural anti-inflammatory prostaglandins, substances naturally derived from the fats of cold water fish and wild game. The decline of these foods in the modern diet may be

Amish Wisdom

The basic Amish treatment program for asthma includes eliminating all refined foods—such as sugar, flour, soft drinks, homogenized milk, coffee, black tea, and chocolate—from the diet. Prudent avoidance of airborne allergens is also a customary treatment of asthma among the Amish.

contributing to the increased incidence of asthma. The body can make these substances from certain vegetable oils, but the process is much more complex and can be inhibited by deficiencies of magnesium, zinc, vitamin B_6 or vitamin C—all common deficiencies in the modern American diet. Science has linked each of these deficiencies—as well as the reduced consumption of cold water fish—to asthma, but the evidence is not strong enough to implicate a single deficiency in all cases. Modern science has also demonstrated that increased salt consumption increases (and reduced salt consumption decreases) the severity of asthma. Although controversial, the industrialization of agriculture and food processing over the last few decades may have contributed to the increased incidence of asthma by exacerbating these deficiencies or excesses. Charles Cropley, a naturopathic physician in Colorado, recently described his dietary regimen for patients with asthma: "Nothing out of a can, nothing out of a box."

If you suffer from asthma, you might want to consider the folk remedies below. After all, these remedies have helped the many generations before us breathe a little easier.

Remedies

LICORICE: Licorice root has long been used to treat coughs and bronchial problems in many cultures throughout the world. It has expectorant properties and also contains anti-inflammatory constituents similar to steroids, although much weaker. Licorice is not so effective in treating an acute asthma attack, but daily use over a long period of time may reduce the body's tendency to overreact to allergens.

☞ DIRECTIONS: Cut 1 ounce of licorice root into slices, cover with 1 quart of boiling water, and steep for 24 hours. Strain and drink 1 or 2 cups a day. Licorice can cause high blood pressure and salt imbalances if taken for long periods. Don't take the above doses if you already have high blood pressure, and don't continue to take the herb in any case for longer than six weeks. (Note that real licorice is not a common ingredient in United States candy. Instead, anise oil is substituted, which has a similar taste.)

MORMON TEA: Mormon tea, the common name for a variety of plants in the *Ephedra* genus, was used as a decongestant for allergies in western American folk medicine among

Emetic Therapy and Asthma

A popular treatment for asthma from the last century was to use an emetic—a substance that induces vomiting. Some herbs were used for this purpose. More often, smaller doses were taken to simply produce expectoration of mucus. The principle of "emetic in large dose but expectorant in small dose" applied to dozens of herbs, including ipecac, bloodroot, and mustard seed. There is no scientific evidence supporting the effectiveness of these herbs in treating asthma, however, possibly due to the difficulty in accurately measuring expectoration.

American Indians, Hispanics, and settlers from the eastern states. A more potent Asian relative called ma huang is used in the same way in traditional Chinese medicine.

The medicinal constituents involved are ephedrine and pseudoephedrine, which also appear in over-the-counter allergy medicines. The American ephedra species do not contain reliable amounts of these constituents. Ma huang and ephedrine-containing drug combinations have been responsible for a number of deaths in the United States in recent years, but generally not when taken as allergy medications. Weight-loss formulas and pep pills sometimes contain ma huang or ephedrine. In this form they are consumed in much larger amounts than in allergy medications and present a greater risk of side effects. Ephedra is contraindicated in heart disease, hypertension, thyroid conditions, prostate disease, anxiety, pregnancy, and concurrent use of pharmaceutical drugs, except with approval of your physician. Mormon tea itself is not usually available in health food stores, but ma huang often is.

☞ DIRECTIONS: Cover 1 teaspoon of Chinese ephedra with 1 cup of boiling water. Let steep ten minutes. Drink the full cup when suffering an acute asthma attack. Prepare the tea ahead of time and keep it in a sealed container in the refrigerator.

GARLIC: Garlic (*Allium sativum*) has long been used to treat bronchial problems in many cultures. Like many of the other herbs used to treat asthma, garlic acts as an expectorant in low doses and an emetic in higher doses, especially if taken on an empty stomach. The Seventh Day Adventists use garlic in the following way to treat an acute asthma attack.

☞ DIRECTIONS: Take 2 cloves of garlic and crush well. Mix in 2 cups of hot water (105°F). Add a pinch of salt. Drink 1 cup rapidly. (Though this remedy may induce vomiting, it may also abort the asthma attack.) Then drink a second cup, which will usually stay down.

Also, you can try simmering the garlic in water for twenty minutes. (This destroys some of the irritating substances that cause nausea.) This treatment came from the 12th century German mystic Hildegarde von Bingen.

MUSTARD SEED: An old New England remedy calls for 1 teaspoon of mustard seed (*Brassica spp.*), taken morning and evening, in the form of a tea or soup. Mustard contains irritating and expectorant sulfur-containing compounds. Like garlic, it can induce vomiting in larger doses and was used for this purpose by the Eclectic physicians of the late 19th and early 20th centuries in cases of narcotic poisoning.

☞ DIRECTIONS: Crush and moisten the mustard seeds well in order to release the constituents. Let the freshly crushed mustard seeds sit in a warm soup or tea for ten to fifteen minutes before drinking. Take two to three times a day.

Jimsonweed

Here's a folk remedy to avoid. Jimsonweed (*Datura stramonium*) was used to treat acute asthma attacks by many groups throughout the United States, including American Indians, New Englanders, Indiana farmers, and settlers in the American Southwest. Jimsonweed seeds were smoked in a pipe or cigarette to calm an acute attack.

Hyoscyamine and scopolamine, two alkaloid constituents of the plant, are proven bronchodilators, and they also dry the secretions of the mucous membranes. The plant is so powerful that some individuals can receive a medicinal dose by simply touching the leaves or inhaling its fragrance, however. High doses can cause temporary psychosis and nightmarish, fearful hallucinations—hence its common names "Devil-weed" and "Loco-weed." The plant or seeds may be fatally poisonous if eaten and should never be kept within reach of children.

DAISY BLOSSOMS: White daisy blossoms (*Chrysanthemum leucanthemum*) were an early traditional asthma remedy in the eastern United States. By the turn of the 20th century, this plant had become a standard medical treatment of the Eclectic physicians.

☞ DIRECTIONS: Take 4 ounces of white daisy blossoms and crush them well. Pour 1 pint of boiling water over them. Steep for one hour and strain. You can take 2 to 3 tablespoons, two to three times a day.

HONEY: Honey has been used in traditional Chinese medicine for more than two thousand years. It is used to treat conditions ranging from asthma, cough, and chronic bronchitis to stomachache, constipation, chronic sinus congestion, canker sores, and burns. To cure a cough, a simple folk remedy from China recommends drinking a tea consisting of hot water and a tablespoon of honey. (This treatment probably isn't strong enough to treat an asthma attack, but it might help thin mucus and prevent congestion.) Expectorant syrups made from honey or sugar are widespread throughout the folk traditions of the world. In the United States, honey syrups appear in the folk medicine of New England, Appalachia, and the Southwest.

GARLIC AND HONEY:
Some syrups combine the healthy benefits of both garlic and honey. Such syrups appear in the folk traditions of New England and the Southwest.

☞ DIRECTIONS: Place 8 ounces of peeled and sliced garlic in 1 pint of boiling water. Let soak for 10 to 12 hours, keeping the water warm, but not boiling. Strain and add 2 pounds of honey. Bottle the mixture. Take 1 teaspoon of the mixture when you're congested.

MULLEIN AND HONEY:
You can use the mullein plant to make an asthma syrup, too. Mullein (Verbascum thapsus) came from Europe to North America with the European colonists and is now naturalized throughout the United States and Canada. Its use as a cough medicine was quickly adopted by various Indian tribes, including the Mohegan, Delaware, Cherokee, Creek, and Navaho. The Penobscot, Potawatomi, and Iroquois used mullein specifically to treat asthma. It was an official medicine in the *United States Pharmacopoeia* from 1888 to 1936. Today, it is an approved medicine for treating coughs in Germany.

☞ DIRECTIONS: Place ½ pound of mullein leaves in a 1-quart jar. Fill the jar with boiling water and let cool to room temperature. Strain. Add honey to the tea until it is the consistency of syrup. Take 1 tablespoon of the syrup when suffering an asthma attack.

NETTLE AND HONEY: This home remedy comes from German immigrants who settled in the New York area. Nettle juice (*Urtica dioica, Urtica urens*) and nettle syrups may still be purchased in Germany today. American physicians of the 19th and early 20th centuries also used nettle to treat some types of allergic conditions. Nettle is an unusually mineral-rich plant. An ounce of the dried herb contains more than two-thirds of the minimum daily requirement of magnesium, which is a frequently deficient mineral in asthma patients.

☞ DIRECTIONS: Take ½ pint of nettle juice, boil it, remove the scum from the pot, and mix the re-

Sweating

A common folk medical treatment of the 19th century was to induce sweating. In *Home Remedies: Hydrotherapy, Massage, Charcoal, and Other Simple Treatments*, co-author Calvin Thrash, M.D., a contemporary teacher and advocate of the Seventh Day Adventist school of natural medicine, writes, "Anything that increases perspiration of the skin will encourage increased activity of the mucous membranes."

Mucous secretions become thick in asthma. When an individual sweats, however, the belief is that the flow of mucus will increase. The increased flow thins the secretions and makes them flow more easily, helping to relieve difficult breathing. Sweating practices are contraindicated in patients who are thirsty or dehydrated, a caution probably overlooked in the 19th century traditions to the detriment of the patient. On this topic, Thomsonian herbalist George Letsum made a play on his name: "First I pukes 'em, then I sweats 'em, and if they dies, then I lets 'em."

maining juice with an equal part of honey. Take 1 tablespoonful in the morning and evening.

FOOT BATH AND TEA: A Seventh Day Adventist treatment for asthma is to induce sweating by putting the feet in warm water and drinking a tea made of catnip *(Napeta cataria)* or pennyroyal *(Hedeoma pulegioides)*. Catnip and pennyroyal are both diaphoretics—they bring circulation to the skin and produce sweating. Don't use this treatment during pregnancy, however; both these herbs promote menstruation. (See sidebar, "Sweating," page 60, for other important contraindications.)

☞ DIRECTIONS: Fill a bathtub or a smaller tub with hot water. Put the feet in the water while drinking the hot tea. (This treatment is contraindicated in diabetics, however, because the feet might become burned.)

To make the tea, place 1 ounce of catnip or pennyroyal leaves in a 1-quart jar and cover with boiling water. Cover the jar tightly and let steep for ten to fifteen minutes. Strain and drink.

❦ Bites and Stings ❦

When bees, wasps, scorpions, and snakes attack humans, it's usually because we threatened them or their living space. On the other hand, insects such as mosquitoes, biting flies, ticks, chiggers, and fleas are predatory pests that view humans as good opportunities for a bite to eat. Their bites are more likely to be itchy than painful. With any bite or sting, the species' venom, or sometimes the tiny insect itself, penetrates the barriers of the body. The combination of the effects of the poison and the body's attempt to eliminate it can cause pain, swelling, or itching near the bite site.

Most bites and stings are not a serious medical concern, but there are a few exceptions. In some people, the stings of bees, wasps, and hornets can cause an allergic reaction called anaphylactic shock. Any shortness of breath or swelling in the airway after a sting is a medical emergency requiring immediate attention. Tick bites can cause Lyme disease or Rocky Mountain spotted fever. Bites of the black widow spider and brown recluse spider can also cause serious medical symptoms; any reaction following a spider bite requires medical attention.

The bites of the poisonous snakes in North America are not usually life threatening to healthy adults. Of about 8,000 such bites in the United States each year, fewer than 15 cause fatalities; the deaths occur mostly in children and the elderly. The illness from a poisonous snake bite can be quite severe, however, and should be treated as a medical emergency. Any snake bite can cause an infected puncture wound, which requires careful cleaning and medical attention. The *Centruroides exilicauda* scorpion, native to Arizona, New Mexico, and the California side of the Colorado River, is the only North American scorpion that can cause serious illness or death. The folk remedies here are for normal itches and pains associated with bites and stings, not for complications caused by Lyme disease, anaphylactic shock, or snake bites.

Remedies

MINTS: American Indian tribes have used various species of mint for the relief and prevention of insect bites. For example, peppermint *(Mentha piperita)* contains camphor, which is cooling to the skin and helps to relieve itching.

☞ DIRECTIONS: Place 1 ounce of peppermint leaf in a 1-quart canning jar and cover with boiling water. Seal the jar tightly and let stand until the water cools to room temperature. Apply to mosquito bites or other itchy areas with a cloth. Reapply as desired.

PENNYROYAL: Early American colonists introduced European pennyroyal to North America, but found the Indians were already using American pennyroyal *(Hedeoma pulegioides)*. The herb was used by American Indians to prevent deer tick bites. In the *Frank C. Brown Collection of North Carolina Folklore,* a North Carolina source says: "Pennyroyal beaten on the legs will keep insects away." Pennyroyal contains eleven separate constituents with identified insect-repellent properties.

☞ DIRECTIONS: Purchase the essential oil of pennyroyal. Put 8 to 10 drops in some almond oil, mix, and apply—especially around the ankles, neck, and scalp—to repel ticks and other insects.

TOBACCO: The Mayan Indians moistened the leaves of wild tobacco *(Nicotiana rustica, N. glauca)* with saliva and applied the leaves to a bite or sting. The Six Nations, a league of Indians that extended from the Hudson River to Lake Erie, also used tobacco to treat insect bites. Using tobacco in this manner later passed into Appalachian folk medicine, where tobacco poultices are still used today to treat bee, hornet, yellow jacket, and wasp stings as well as spider bites. In the folk medicine of the Southwest, a strong tobacco tea is applied to tick bites to help draw the tick out. Physicians of the last century also supported tobacco's antiseptic qualities: They

Louisiana Snake Magic

Louisiana folklore recalls the magical traditions of Africa and the voudon. A book of Louisiana folk remedies suggests that, if bitten by a snake near water, you need to beat the snake back to the water. Then, you must dip the bitten area of your body into the water. If you do this, the snake will die instead of you. Another folk remedy for treating snakebites suggests cutting open a black hen, and while she is still jumping, holding her over the bite. When the hen has stopped fluttering, the poison will be gone. Specialized "snake doctors" in rural Louisiana would also suck on snakebites, attempting to remove the poison. All these remedies seemed to work—because most people recover from a snakebite with nothing more than a little bed rest.

used tobacco ointments and tobacco poultices to treat skin conditions.

☞ DIRECTIONS: Mix tobacco from cigarettes, cigars, chewing tobacco, or snuff with water and apply directly to a bite or sting. Leave the mixture on as long as you like.

PLANTAIN LEAVES:Plantain *(Plantago spp.),* the common four-leafed weed that grows in lawns and around sidewalks throughout the country, was once called "White Man's Foot-print" by the eastern American Indians because it came to this country with the European immigrants and spread wherever they went. Various tribes quickly adopted the plant as a medicine for treating bites, stings, and minor wounds. The Six Nations (see remedy, Tobacco, page 63) used the plant specifically to treat spider bites. Plantain leaves are still used today in the folk medicine of Indiana, North Carolina, and the Southwest. Plantain's chemical constituents may explain its ability to soothe pain and promote wound healing: It contains at least fifteen constituents with identified anti-inflammatory properties, seventeen with bactericidal properties, six analgesics, and five antiseptics. It also contains a constituent that promotes cell proliferation and tissue healing.

☞ DIRECTIONS: Crush a small handful of fresh plantain leaves and apply locally to bites and stings. Applied externally, the plant stimulates and cleanses the skin and encourages wounds to heal faster. You can apply fresh leaves every fifteen to twenty minutes. Leave on as long as desired.

GARLIC AND ONIONS: Cultivated garlic *(Allium sativum)*, onions *(Allium cepa)*, and their wild relatives have appeared in the medical records of all major civilizations since ancient times. Both garlic and onion have been used as antidotes to the poisons of bites and stings, taken internally or applied externally to the bite area. In North American folk medicine, the Amish and residents of Indiana apply crushed garlic or raw onions directly to snake, scorpion, or insect bites. Garlic and onion have also been used for this purpose in New England, in the Southwest, and in Chinatowns of the West Coast.

Both garlic and onions contain broad spectrum antibiotic and anti-inflammatory substances that can disinfect and soothe a bite or sting.

☞ DIRECTIONS: Crush a clove of garlic and mix it with a little water or saliva. Apply directly to the bite area. Also, you can blend up 3 cloves of garlic in 1 cup of wine, and let the mixture sit overnight. Wash any infected bites or stings hourly with the wine mixture the next day. Place a thick slice of onion over the bite area. Leave on as long as you like.

VINEGAR: In the folklore of New England, rural

Indiana, the parts of the American Southwest, and among Gypsies and the Amish, a vinegar wash is sometimes recommended for treating bites and stings.

☞ DIRECTIONS: Use undiluted vinegar as a wash to stop itching or to relieve the pain of stings. Also, you can try this Gypsy recipe: Take a handful of thyme *(Thymus vulgaris)* and seal it in a bottle of vinegar for one cycle of the moon, in the sun if possible. Shake the bottle every morning and evening. Then, after an additional half cycle of the moon, crush seven garlic cloves and add them to the bottle. At the end of the second lunar cycle, strain and bottle the liquid. Use as a wash for itchy or infected bites.

CHARCOAL: A charcoal poultice is a medical treatment of the Seventh Day Adventists for insect and snake bites. Charcoal has strong drawing properties and is sometimes taken internally to neu-tralize ingested poisons in the gut.

☞ DIRECTIONS: Wet as much crushed charcoal as you need to cover the injured area. Place the charcoal directly over the area and cover with a clean cloth. Replace the poultice every ten to fifteen minutes until relief is obtained.

BAKING SODA: Applying baking soda paste to spider bites and bee stings to relieve pain or itching is a folk remedy still used today in North Carolina, New England, the South-west, and among the Amish. This remedy re-portedly reduces swelling and pain if applied to the skin immediately after the bite has occurred.

☞ DIRECTIONS: Moisten baking soda with water and apply the mix-ture directly to the af-fected area. You can also use vinegar to moisten the baking soda, or mix the baking soda with equal parts of salt and add water to form a paste. Leave on for as long as desired.

CLAY: Using clay or mud-packs to treat bee and wasp stings seems to be a universal folk remedy. In North America, it appears in the folk literature of southern blacks, Canadians, New Englanders, New Yorkers, North Carolinians, the Aztec Indians of Mexico, and contemporary Hispanics in Texas and New Mexico. Some people believe the clay works by literally drawing the toxins out of the body.

☞ DIRECTIONS: Apply mud or cold clay (any kind of clay soil or cosmetic clay will do) to the sting area to relieve pain and reduce swelling. When the clay dries, apply new clay. Repeat this as long as necessary.

KEROSENE: A remedy from contemporary southern Appalachians is to apply kerosene to bee stings to relieve pain and swelling.

☞ DIRECTIONS: Wash the sting area with kerosene, or soak a cloth in kerosene and apply it to the area as a poultice. Kerosene itself can be irritating, so don't keep the poultice in place for more than twenty to thirty minutes.

❦ Bladder and ❧ Kidney Infections

▨ ▨ ▨

The urinary system includes those organs of the body that produce or eliminate urine. By controlling urine flow, the system maintains proper water balance in the body. Changes in urine and urinary habits that do not seem to have an obvious cause may be symptoms of disease. An accurate diagnosis by a physician is the first step to proper treatment.

Most pathological conditions of the kidney and bladder are not appropriate for self-treatment with folk or home remedies. Even bladder infections, the least serious of common urinary tract conditions, require a diagnosis to rule out sexually transmitted diseases or more serious kidney involvement. Most of the folk remedies below for treating urinary tract infections work in the same way as conventional treatment recommendations, however. For example, drinking adequate water to wash out bacteria is a standard procedure in both folk and conventional medicine for treating urinary tract infections.

Most of the folk remedies in this section use herbs with mild diuretic properties. These herbs increase the flow of urine through the urinary tract, helping to wash out irritating substances. In Germany, the use of such mild diuretics is called "flushing out therapy"; in that country, the therapy is a routine conventional treatment for bladder infections and stone prevention. Research has shown that mild diuretics increase urination and reduce joint swelling. Thus, mild natural diuretics are also used in Germany for treating the swollen joints of arthritis.

An important restriction on the use of herbal diuretics, however, is in cases of edema resulting from heart, kidney, or liver disease. (The condition was once known as "dropsy.") Edema requires careful medical attention—and properly monitored doses of diuretics. Although some folk remedies were once used to treat edema, during the 20th century, modern medical science has discovered much safer and more effective treatments for the condition.

The remedies in this section are found in many cultures throughout the world. In fact, most of these remedies would be included in classes on urinary tract herbs in medical schools in Germany, where doctors and pharmacists are required by law to receive training in medical herbalism.

A topic not included in this section is urinary difficulties due to prostate problems. Any obstructive problems of the urinary tract due to enlargement of the prostate require conventional medical attention to determine the cause.

Remedies

STINGING NETTLE: The Chippewa and Sioux Indian tribes used the leaves of the stinging nettle plant (*Urtica spp.*) as a mild diuretic for flushing out the urinary tract. It is used the same way today by Gypsies in Europe. Stinging nettle is also used as a diuretic by contemporary professional medical herbalists in North America and Europe and is an approved medical treatment for bladder infections in

Germany. Besides having a mild diuretic effect, nettle is highly nutritious. An ounce of the leaves contains a large portion of the daily requirement for several minerals.

☞ DIRECTIONS: Simmer 1 ounce of stinging nettle leaf in 1 quart of water for twenty minutes. Strain and drink 3 to 4 cups a day for a week or two.

CORN SILK: Corn silk (*Zea mays*), the hairy projections from the end of an ear of corn, was introduced as a medicine to the Western world after the European conquest of Mexico, Central America, and South America. Corn, native to those areas, is now cultivated not only in the Americas, but as far away as Africa, India, and China. Corn silk tea was used as a diuretic by American Indians in the conquered regions and is now used in the same way in folk traditions throughout North America and Europe. It has even entered into formal Chinese

Kidney Stones

A myth perpetuated in many modern herbals and collections of folk remedies is that certain herbs or foods will "dissolve stones." Kidney stones are formed when certain salts become too concentrated in the urine. Once formed, they do not readily dissolve back into the urine, however, and must either pass down the urinary tract or be broken up or dissolved by conventional medical means. Certain individuals, sometimes referred to in conventional medicine as "stone formers," tend to suffer repeat attacks of kidney stones. For them, the best treatment for kidney stones is prevention, which involves drinking plenty of water to dilute the urine. Drinking large amounts of fluids, particularly at night, reduces urine concentration so that stones cannot form.

medical traditions, where it is called "yu mi shu." It is often prescribed as a diuretic by medical herbalists of Europe, North America, and Australia.

☞ DIRECTIONS: Fill a 1-quart jar one-third full of fresh corn silk. Pour enough boiling water to fill the jar, cover, and let cool to room temperature. Strain and drink the quart in 4 doses during the day for seven to ten days.

JOE-PYE WEED: Queen of the meadow (*Eupatorium purpureum, Eupatorium maculatum*) was used medicinally by eastern American Indians, including the Cherokee and Mohawk tribes, before the arrival of European colonists. An Indian healer named Joe Pye reportedly used it to treat a group of colonists suffering from typhoid fever, and the survivors of the epidemic named the plant in honor of him—thus, Joe-Pye weed. It also has been called "gravel root" because of its prominent use as a treatment for kidney stones.

Queen of the meadow was used by Eclectic physicians from about 1848 until the group's demise in the 1940s. The Eclectics preferred Queen of the meadow over some other diuretic plants because of its non-irritating effects. One of the Eclectic physicians, Harvey Felter, M.D., stated in a turn-of-the-century medical book, *King's American Dispensatory*, that the herb was effective in treating kidney stones for two reasons—first, because it increased the flow of urine, preventing stone formation or washing out existing stones, and second, it reduced inflammation and pain in the urinary tract. Felter disputed the common myth that the plant could dissolve kidney stones that had already formed, however.

Queen of the meadow is recommended in the folklore of North Carolina residents for treating or preventing painful urinary tract conditions. The plant is still prescribed as a diuretic for bladder infections and kidney stones by professional medical herbalists in North America, although it has not been used in North American or European conventional medicine since the time of the Eclectics (see sidebar, "Eclectic Medicine," page 25).

☞ DIRECTIONS: Add ½ ounce of queen of the meadow to a pint of water. (Queen of the meadow may be sold in your herb shop under the name "gravel root.") Cover and simmer for twenty minutes. Let cool to room temperature. Drink 2 to 3 cups a day, while also drinking plenty of water.

WATERMELON: Watermelon seed tea (*Citrullus vulgaris*) is a folk diuretic mentioned in the literature of Indiana and North Carolina. It is also recommended by the Amish and the Seventh Day Adventists, the latter being a religious movement that advocates natural remedies *continued on page 74*

continued on page 74

Simple Beliefs on Bedwetting

※ ※ ※

Childhood can be a difficult time in any culture, and many folk remedies are aimed at curing common problems for children. One concern is bedwetting. Sometimes bedwetting can be a symptom of infection or other physical difficulty. Other times, children just don't wake up when they need to urinate. Not only is bedwetting messy, but it can be embarrassing to both child and parent. Some of the folk remedies used to cure it, however, are even more embarrassing. For example, draping the wet sheet over the child's head and making him stand outside in the sun until it dries is one recommended remedy!

Some say a child playing with hot ashes before going to bed at night will suffer the affliction. But you can cure him of bedwetting by heating a brick and having the child urinate on it.

It is believed that what you do with the umbilical cord when a child is born can cause or prevent a child from

Mouse Tea?

Some of the most peculiar cures for bedwetting use rats or mice. Boiling a mouse for a tea is one method. Roasting or frying a mouse or rat and having the child eat part of it, sometimes in a sandwich or pie, is another treatment. The strangest use is to wrap a mouse in a cloth and bite off its head, then tie the cloth, with the head in it, around the child's neck—and leave it there for several days. With all the diseases we can catch from rodents and their fleas, these treatments could make a child, or you, very sick!

becoming a bedwetter. Laying an umbilical cord down will cause the child to be a bedwetter. Some say that if you burn the "navel string" the child won't wet the bed.

Belief in the curative power of corpses is widespread. So is the idea that burying something in a grave will cure the person associated with the item. Some people have even tried to get a child to urinate in an open grave to cure bedwetting. Another related remedy involves putting a bottle of the child's urine in a grave before the grave is closed up. Put a small hole in the bottle's cork so the urine can drip out. When it does, the bedwetting will be cured.

Seeds and teas are commonly used in folk remedies. Feeding a child watermelon seeds or pumpkin seeds is said to cure bedwetting. Both corn silk and gum bark teas have also been tried. A rare parent or two has even squeezed the urine from the sheets, mixed it with milk and sugar, and made the child drink that! This remedy could actually poison a child and lead to much worse problems than bedwetting!

and alternative medicine. Watermelon seed was also used as a diuretic by Eclectic physicians during the last century. Today, it is not commonly found in medical herbalism, probably because it is not always available in herb stores.

☞ DIRECTIONS: Place a handful of fresh watermelon seeds in the bottom of a 1-pint jar and fill with boiling water. Let cool to room temperature. Strain and drink a pint of the tea each day for seven to ten days.

PUMPKIN SEEDS: Another diuretic often mentioned in folk literature is pumpkin seeds (*Cucurbita pepo*). The folk traditions of New England, Indiana, and Louisiana all suggest taking a few pumpkin seeds to promote urination. The Eclectic physicians of the last century followed the practice until the group's demise in the 1940s.

Contemporary German physicians use pumpkin seed preparations to treat difficult urination that accompanies enlarged prostate (when prostate cancer as a cause has been ruled out). Two constituents in pumpkin seeds, adenosine and cucurbitacin, both have diuretic properties.

☞ DIRECTIONS: Crush a handful of fresh pumpkin seeds and place in the bottom of a 1-pint jar. Fill with boiling water. Let cool to room temperature. Strain and drink a pint of the tea each day.

Also, you can eat pumpkin seeds according to taste. It is best to remove the shells and eat them with little or no salt.

WATER: The most obvious diuretic to increase the flow of urine is water. Simply drinking

Sugar

The Spanish Gypsy folk healer Pilar, the source of the remedies in a book called *Gypsy Folk Medicine* by Wanja von Hausen, recommends against adding sugar or honey to diuretic teas used for treating urinary tract infections. This is sound advice, from a medical point of view, for any infection, actually. Clinical studies have shown that about 2 ounces of sugar—the amount in the average soft drink—depresses the activity of the immune system's white blood cells by about 40 percent. Cranberry juices sweetened with sugar should be avoided for this reason. Although a clinical trial showed that sugar-sweetened cranberry juice does help prevent bladder infections, it is likely that the juice may be more effective without the sugar.

plenty of water—6 to 8 glasses a day—can increase urine flow, dilute the urine to prevent stone formation, and wash out bacteria that may cause infections. Some of the benefits of the mild diuretic teas used by physicians in Germany and by professional herbalists in North America come from the tea's increased volume of water. German physician R.F. Weiss, M.D., suggested that individuals who are prone to forming stones should, one day a week, consume a quart and a half of water rapidly (within fifteen minutes) to wash out any tiny stones that may be forming.

☞ DIRECTIONS: Drink 6 to 8 glasses of water a day. Or, one day a week, drink 6 glasses of water in rapid succession, within fifteen minutes, to flush out the urinary tract.

CRANBERRY JUICE: One of the most famous folk remedies for bladder infections—widely followed today throughout

Demulcent Herbs

Demulcents are a class of herbs that soothe irritated mucous membranes. They have a slimy mucous-like texture when mixed with water. The demulcents marshmallow (*Althea officinalis*), slippery elm (*Ulmus fulva*), and mullein leaf (*Verbascum thapsus*) all have been used in North American folk traditions to soothe urinary tract inflammation. The demulcents are often combined with diuretic herbs and taken as teas.

North America—is to drink cranberry juice. This remedy is especially well known in the folk medicine of New England.

This remedy, which has been studied in modern clinical trials, has been found to be effective in preventing, but not treating, bladder infections. A study conducted at the Brigham and Women's Hospital in Boston, and published in the prestigious *Journal of the American Medical Association* in 1994, found that consumption of about 12 ounces of commercial cranberry juice each day for a month reduced bacterial counts in the lower urinary tracts of elderly women. Several other trials have shown similar results. (Using cranberry juice as a preventive may be very useful to bedridden elders, who are at higher risk for bladder infections.)

Constituents in the cranberry juice help to prevent bacteria from sticking to the walls of the urinary tract, making the bacteria easier to flush out. Once the infection is underway, however, and the bacteria have set up shop, the cranberry juice is not of much use.

☞ DIRECTIONS: Obtain a sugar-free cranberry juice or juice concentrate from a health food store. (The brands in supermarkets contain enough sugar to depress the activity of the immune system.) Drink 8 to 12 ounces of the juice a day to prevent recurring bladder infections.

PARSLEY: The ancient Egyptians, Greeks, and Romans all used parsley *(Petroselinum crispum)* as a diuretic. The practice continues today both by Gypsies and in the folk tradition of New England. Parsley, which originated in the eastern Mediterranean region, was introduced to England in the year 1548, and, within a hundred years, it was recommended in British medical herbals for use as a diuretic in cases of severe edema (dropsy).

Although edema is now treated with conventional medicine, parsley can still be used to remedy other conditions. Parsley is approved by the German government for use as a mild diuretic and for treatment of bladder infections. For safety's sake, use parsley root rather than parsley seeds, parsley juice, or parsley leaves. (Parsley seeds can stimulate uterine contractions or irritate the kidneys. Parsley juice can also stimulate uterine contractions and should thus be avoided during pregnancy. And, although parsley leaves are nutritious, they do not contain much of the diuretic constituents of the plant.) The following formula is a modification of a Gypsy diuretic formula used for urinary tract infections and kidney stones.

☞ DIRECTIONS: Take a handful of parsley roots and cut them into small pieces. Place them in 1 quart of water, bring to a boil, and simmer for ten to fifteen minutes. Remove from the heat and stir in a handful of rose blossoms. Steep, covered, for ten minutes. Strain and drink 5 to 7 cups of the tea during the course of a day for seven to ten days. Do not use in excessive amounts. Do not use during pregnancy and lactation.

BURDOCK: Burdock *(Arctium spp.)* has been used since ancient times as a mild diuretic. The Iroquois Indians used the root for this purpose. In 17th century Great Britain, the plant's seeds were used specifically for treating the bladder and kidney stones.

In Germany, burdock is commonly used in contemporary medical practice, even though a review by the German government failed to find adequate clinical research to justify its use. However, in 1994, animal research in Spain demonstrated that, while burdock root teas did lower the risk factors for kidney stones and kidney infections, the effect was mild. And, although burdock is widely used in contemporary North American professional herbalism, its most common use in this country is as a "blood cleanser," not a diuretic.

☞ DIRECTIONS: Place 1 ounce of burdock root in 1 quart of water in a pot and simmer, covered, for twenty minutes. Let cool to room temperature. Strain and drink the quart of tea throughout the day.

Do this for up to three weeks.

BUCHU: The Hottentot tribe of southern Africa first acquainted Europeans with the use of buchu *(Barosma betulina)*. In 1821, it was imported to England. By 1840, it appeared in the *United States Pharmacopoeia* as an official medicine; it remained listed in following editions until 1940. It was used for treating urinary tract infections by all schools of medicine during that period. (The Eclectic physicians cautioned that the plant's oils could further irritate those urinary tract infections that are accompanied by burning or stinging pain, however.) The plant's constituents are probably its aromatic peppermint-like oils. Buchu is used by conventional doctors in Germany as a mild diuretic and for treatment of bladder infections.

☞ DIRECTIONS: Place ½ ounce of buchu leaves and ½ ounce of marshmallow root *(Althea offici-*

nalis) in 1 quart of water. Cover the pot and simmer on the lowest heat for thirty to forty minutes. Allow to cool to room temperature. Strain and drink 1-ounce doses three to four times a day for seven to ten days.

WATER IMMERSION: The Seventh Day Adventists recommend sitting in a hot tub to promote urination. According to clinical research over the last ten years, full water immersion (up to the neck) can indeed produce this effect. (Apparently, the increased water pressure on the body promotes increased excretion of urine.) Research shows the same effect regardless of whether hot, cold, or neutral-temperature water is used.

☞ DIRECTIONS: After drinking 2 to 3 glasses of water, immerse yourself for thirty to forty minutes in a hot tub, swimming pool, or other body of water.

❧ Blood Purifiers ❧ and Blood Builders

❊ ❊ ❊

European and North American folk remedy books from the 18th and 19th centuries make frequent references to foods and herbs that "purify the blood." This concept was also important in conventional and alternative medicine in these centuries and survives today among practitioners of folk medicine. The "blood" in the traditional concept of bad blood did not really refer to the blood at all, but actually to the extracellular fluid that bathes the cells. The blood itself comprises only about five percent of the fluids in the body, while the extracellular fluid makes up about 20 percent. The rest of the body's water lies within the cells.

The composition of the blood is tightly controlled by the physiological mechanisms of the body, so it does not become "bad" in any sense. The extracellular fluid, on the other hand, accumulates the metabolic wastes of all the cells, the waste byproducts of infection and inflammation, and toxic byproducts of poor digestion. An overload of such materials in the extracellular spaces is probably what physicians of the last century referred to as "bad blood." These doctors included such medical conditions as abscesses, arthritis, boils, chronic infection, chronic inflammation, eczema, gangrene, psoriasis, septicemia, skin ulcers, and chronically swollen glands in their list of illnesses arising from "bad blood"

and used "blood purifying" herbal medicines and diets to treat them. In folk medicine, the term "spring tonic" is equivalent to "blood purifier" in 19th century medicine. People felt the need to use such tonics in the spring—after months of reduced activity and a lack of fresh fruits and vegetables during the winter.

The concept of bad blood has been abandoned completely in modern medicine, due to advances in the science of physiology and to a lack of clinical trials of most of the herbs formerly used. If you see references to such terms in books of folk or herbal medicine, know that they do not apply to true blood diseases in the modern sense. But the concept of blood purification is alive and well in contemporary professional medical herbalism in North America, Great Britain, and Australia, even if the term itself is not accurate. Five of the ten most often prescribed herbs by professional

Good for Molasses

New Englanders, Indiana farmers, and the people of Appalachia have long used molasses as a "blood builder," either alone or added to blood-purifying teas and foods. Why? Molasses is one of the most mineral-dense foods available to us. Two tablespoons of blackstrap molasses, the most concentrated form, contain 340 milligrams of calcium, 6.5 milligrams of iron, 85 milligrams of magnesium, 1000 milligrams of potassium, .75 milligram of copper, and 1 milligram of manganese, all significant portions of the recommended dietary allowance.

herbalists in these countries, recorded in a 1994 poll, were traditional blood purifiers.

The actions of the herbs are varied. They include immune stimulants such as echinacea and garlic; circulatory stimulants such as cayenne; bitter liver-stimulating herbs such as dandelion, yellow dock, and goldenseal; diuretics like nettle; and sweat-inducing herbs such as burdock and boneset.

Remedies

BURDOCK: Burdock root (*Arctium lappa, Arctium minus*) has long been a universal "blood purifier" among North American peoples. Its medicinal value was noted by the ancient Greeks; it arrived in North America via the European colonists. Burdock's medicinal use was rapidly adopted by the Mohegan, Delaware, Chippewa, Omaha, Potawatomi, and Cherokee Indian tribes. It is used today in the folk medicine of Pennsylvania Germans, the Amish, Indiana farmers, and residents throughout Appalachia. Burdock has become naturalized throughout North America except in Texas and Alaska and parts of Canada.

Burdock was an official medicine in the *United States Pharmacopoeia* from 1831 to 1842, and again from 1851 to 1916. It was recommended as a diuretic, mild laxative, and treatment for skin ailments. Modern scientific studies show that burdock root has anti-inflammatory properties, slightly opposes the tendency of the blood to clot, and scavenges destructive free radicals from the blood.

☞ DIRECTIONS: Simmer 1 ounce of burdock root in 1 pint of water for twenty minutes. Strain when cool. Add 3 or 4 tablespoons of molasses. Drink the entire contents over the course of a day. Repeat daily for one to two weeks.

ECHINACEA: Echinacea *(Echinacea angustifolia, Echinacea purpurea)* was used extensively by the Northern Plains Indians to treat burns and wounds as well as the bites of snakes and poisonous insects. Echinacea was adopted by the Eclectic medical profession in the mid 1800s, and became their most-often prescribed medicine by about 1920. The Eclectics, a group of M.D.s who primarily used herbs as medicines, classified the plant as a blood purifier and used it to treat life-threatening blood infections. German physicians began using the plant by the 1830s, and, in that country, it remains a frequently-prescribed medicine today. Folklorists have also discovered the use of echinacea in the folk medicine of the Appalachians in northern Georgia, but its use undoubtedly arrived there in the last century from outside the area.

Echinacea root is used primarily to boost the immune system and help the body fight disease. Besides bolstering several chemical substances that direct immune response, echinacea increases the number and activity of white blood cells, raises the level of interferon (a substance that enhances immune function), increases production of substances the body produces to fight cancer, and helps remove pollutants from the lungs. Many studies support echinacea's ability to fend off disease. It is perhaps the best known remedy of the modern folk herbal.

Echinacea is not effective as a tea for immune-building properties, but must be taken as a tincture, or, as in the case of the Plains Indians, the whole root can be chewed.

☞ DIRECTIONS: Purchase an alcohol tincture of echinacea at a health food store or herb store. To prevent illness, take 1 dropperful three times a day. If you are sick with a cold or flu or feel a cold coming on, take a dropperful mixed with a little warm water every two hours.

To make your own tincture, purchase 1 pound of echinacea root. In a jar, cover the root with grain alcohol or 100 proof liquor. Close the jar tightly. Store in a cool dark place for three weeks, turning or shaking the jar daily. Then strain and store in the refrigerator. Use as directed above.

GARLIC: Garlic *(Allium sativum)* has been prized for millennia, used by the Egyptians, Hebrews, Romans, Greeks, and Chinese. It has appeared in the ancient medical texts of every traditional form of medicine. Garlic is one of the most extensively researched and widely used plants. Its actions are diverse and affect nearly every body system. The herb boasts antibiotic, antifungal, and antiviral properties and is reported to be effective against many influenza strains. Garlic inhibits blood clotting and keeps platelets from clumping, which improves blood flow and reduces the risk of stroke. Its widest known folk use is as a tonic to "ward off" disease or evil.

Because garlic was not native to this country (it may have originated in southern Siberia), Indian tribes in the eastern

An Endangered Species

"Goldenseal is the king and queen of herbs that the Good Lord put in the ground," according to traditional Appalachian herbalist Tommie Bass in *Herbal Medicine Past and Present* (Volume II), by John K. Crellin and Jane Philpott. The Cherokee Indians mixed powdered goldenseal root with bear grease and slathered their bodies to protect themselves from mosquitoes and other insects. Pioneers adapted the herb and used it to treat wounds, rashes, mouth sores, morning sickness, liver and stomach complaints, internal hemorrhaging, depressed appetite, constipation, and urinary and uterine problems.

Goldenseal formerly abounded in the eastern forests of this country, but, due to overharvesting (it takes about five years for the root to get large enough to harvest) and loss of habitat, it was recently declared an endangered species. Goldenseal is contraindicated in acute colds and flu (it can make them worse) and is ineffective when used to mask the presence of drugs in urine specimens. Unfortunately, these are the two most common modern uses, and such misuse is probably contributing to the extinction of the plant.

United States used garlic's native botanical cousin, the onion, as a spring tonic. European immigrants brought their native folk uses of garlic with them, and the garlic plant was ultimately naturalized here. A single clove (not the whole bulb) of garlic a day has shown to have preventive effects against disease.

☞ DIRECTIONS: One of the best ways to consume garlic is to eat it raw. You can eat up to 3 cloves a day. When cooked, the stronger the flavor is, the more medicinal value it has. Alternately, try blending 1 to 3 cloves of garlic in a cup of your favorite juice, warm water, or wine, and let stand covered overnight. Strain and drink the next day, in 3 divided doses, with meals.

CAYENNE PEPPERS: Cayenne peppers *(Capsicum spp.)* were used by the Aztec Indians as a remedy for "bad blood." The practice continues in the folk medicine of the American Southwest, although the usual form of administration is as a seasoning in food. Cayenne peppers are a strong circulatory stimulant and were one of the main remedies of the Thomsonian movement of folk herbalism during the first half of the 19th century. The stimulation of blood circulation to the periphery of the body is presumably how the peppers "purify" those areas where circulation is believed to have stagnated. Because chiles are so heating, they are probably best suited to those individuals with "cold" consti-

tutions—those with cold hands and feet and a tendency to chill easily. Says Dr. William Cook, author of a mid-19th century medical herbal called *The Physio-Medicalist Dispensatory*: "Cayenne is as out of place in a hot constitution as a bonfire on the Fourth of July."

☞ DIRECTIONS: Use chiles freely as a food condiment. Alternately, sprinkle ¼ teaspoon of cayenne powder into 1 cup of warm water and add a little lemon juice. Drink the mixture twenty minutes before meals. Do this three times a day for up to two weeks. Adjust the quantity of the pepper to your taste.

DANDELION: Through their writings, the Arabs were the first to introduce dandelion's *(Taraxacum officinale)* healing and nutritive abilities to the Europeans. By the 16th century, dandelion was considered an important culinary and blood-purifying herb in Europe. The root was recommended to treat liver diseases, such as jaundice and cirrhosis. The remedies requiring the use of dandelion traveled to North America with European immigrants; some eastern American Indian groups also used dandelion for healing purposes. The dandelion has become naturalized in this country throughout temperate regions.

Dandelion was an official medicine in the *United States Pharmacopoeia* from 1831 to 1926, recommended as a diuretic, tonic, and mild laxative. Modern scientific trials show that dandelion acts as a mild diuretic and increases the flow of bile from the liver, and, in one animal trial, it helped to restore depleted immune function.

Dandelion roots contain inulin and levulin, starch-like substances that are easy to digest, as well as a bitter substance (taraxacin) that improves digestion through the stimulation of stomach secretions. Because taraxacin does stimulate these secretions,

however, dandelion is contraindicated if you have heartburn or other kinds of digestive pain.

☞ DIRECTIONS: Eat young spring dandelion greens either raw, or lightly sauteed with olive oil, lemon, and garlic. To make a tea of the root, place 1 ounce of the dried chopped root in 1 pint of water and simmer for twenty minutes. Cool and strain. Drink the pint in 3 doses throughout the day. Do this periodically.

YELLOW DOCK: Yellow dock *(Rumex crispus)* has been used in European medicine since the time of the ancient Greeks as a bitter tonic, laxative, liver stimulant, and dressing for wounds. American Indians used North American species of yellow dock in similar ways. It is still used in folk medicine today by some residents in the Appalachian mountains and in the rural Midwest.

Yellow dock root stimulates intestinal secretions and promotes bile flow, which aids fat digestion and has a light laxative action. Long considered a blood purifier, yellow dock may also be effective in treating a number of conditions that stem from liver dysfunction. (Yellow dock has strong laxative properties, so it should be taken in low doses.) It is contraindicated in pregnancy because the constituents it contains that stimulate the bowels may also stimulate the smooth muscle of the uterus.

☞ DIRECTIONS: Place 2 tablespoons of chopped dried yellow dock root in 1 pint of boiling water. Simmer for twenty minutes. Cool and strain. The dose is 3 tablespoons three times a day. Try the treatment for a week or two.

BEETS: American folk remedies list several sources that mention beet juice as a blood purifier. One source states that only raw beets should be used because cooking them destroys whatever blood cleansing properties are present. The contemporary Amish use beet juice as a "blood builder," sometimes mixed with red grape juice. Beets contain betaine, which has beneficial effects on the liver, and several other constituents with anti-inflammatory and immunostimulant properties. Beets are eaten instead of juiced in Appalachia, however.

☞ DIRECTIONS: Purchase beets (home grown or organically grown) and juice them in a juicer. Drink an 8-ounce glass each day for a few weeks. You can eat beets whole, too.

STINGING NETTLE: In Appalachian folk medicine, nettle (*Urtica dioica*) is a *continued on page 89*

Stopping Blood

Bleeding can be both frightening and dangerous. Even without a full understanding of the circulatory system, you can easily figure out that uncontrolled bleeding can be serious, even life-threatening. Every culture has ways of stopping bleeding.

Putting substances on a cut to stop bleeding is a universal practice. Possibly the most widespread practice is washing minor cuts in cold water, or its ruder cousin, spit. A common practice in the United States is putting spiderwebs over cuts or wounds. The spiderwebs may be reinforced with soot or ashes, which must come from a wood-burning fire. This remedy is believed, however, to cause black scars.

Other widely used materials for treating wounds are axle grease and even fresh horse manure! Putting any of these substances on a cut or wound, except clean water, of course, increases your risk of infection and scarring.

Many remedies to stop bleeding focus on nosebleeds. Some claim that tying a piece of metal on a string and letting it hang down your back is a good way to stop a nosebleed. Another suggested way to stop the bleeding is to chew on a piece of paper or fold it and place it under your upper lip. Still another method is to wear a piece of red yarn or silk thread around your neck.

Of course, there are more technical ways to stop nosebleeds. Pressing a blood vessel behind your ear is one way, for example. A more widespread remedy requires the application of cold water to the top (or back) of the head and the back of the neck. In fact, some people have claimed that applying anything cold to the back of the neck will quickly stop a nosebleed.

traditional spring tonic. It is taken as a tea or tincture after a long winter of sedentary habits and a lack of fresh fruits and vegetables, common in all agrarian communities in regions with cold winters. Preparations are used today in European medicine to treat arthritis and enlarged prostate. Modern research shows that nettle has an anti-inflammatory effect. The herb is also highly nutritious—an ounce of nettle contains more than the minimum daily requirement of calcium, two thirds of the requirement of magnesium, and more than one third of the requirement of potassium.

☞ DIRECTIONS: Place 1 ounce of dried nettle in 1 quart of water and simmer until one third of the liquid is evaporated. Cool and strain. Drink the remaining liquid in 3 divided doses. Also, try this method, told to traditional Appalachian herbalist Tommie Bass by a local American Indian: Place 1 inch of dried nettle in the bottom of a 1-pint bottle and fill the bottle with whiskey. Let the bottle sit for a week, shaking it daily. Then take 1 tablespoon of the mixture three times a day. Take for two to three weeks.

BONESET: Boneset (*Eupatorium perfoliatum*) was without a doubt the most famous of the bitter tonics in the early American colonies. (A bitter tonic was a tonic used to stimulate digestion.) Medical botanists Walter and Memory Lewis, in their book *Medical Botany,* state that boneset "was always found in the well-regulated household."

Boneset earned its name because, as a hot tea, it reportedly cured "breakbone fever," an old term for influenza. It is usually taken as a cold tea in small doses. High doses can induce vomiting; it was used for this purpose by physicians of the 19th century.

☞ DIRECTIONS: To use as a bitter tonic, place 1 tablespoon of dried boneset leaves in a cup and cover with boiling water. Let stand until the water is room temperature. Strain and drink in 3 divided doses during the day, away from meals.

ELDER: The berries and flowers of the black elder *(Sambucus nigra)* have been used as a blood purifier and flu remedy. In British folk herbalism it was taken in the form of elderberry wine. The berries of the North American variety of the plant, *Sambucus canadensis*, were used for the same purposes by the Houma Indians of Louisiana. European settlers brought elderberry plants with them to the American colonies.

Elder was an official medicine in the *United States Pharmacopoeia* from 1820 to 1905. It was recommended as an "alterative," an old medical term for blood purifier. The elderberry that bears blue fruit is perfectly safe to eat, although large quantities of the raw berries can cause some indigestion and act as a laxative. Cooking the berries before eating them cancels this action. The leaves, bark, and root, on the other hand, are slightly toxic and should not be ingested. Don't use the elder plant that bears red berries. This plant is of a different species.

☞ DIRECTIONS: Fill half of a 1-quart pot with elderberries. Add water until the pot is nearly full and bring to a boil. Simmer on the lowest heat until one third of the water has evaporated. Strain and store in the refrigerator. Add 1 teaspoon to a cup of water and drink three times a day. Do this for two to three weeks.

SASSAFRAS: Sassafras *(Sassafras albidum)* was used as a spring tonic in the eastern parts of the United States, throughout New England, among the Pennsylvania Germans, and through Appalachia all the way to northern Georgia and Alabama. Colonists learned the use of sassafras from the Indians. Spanish colonists used it as a universal remedy and shipped samples back to Spain. The plant was considered such an important medicine by colonists in Virginia and Massachusetts that boatloads of it were shipped back to England after the year 1602.

Sassafras has a wide variety of active constituents, several of them with cancer-preventing properties. It also contains the constituent saffrole, which has been found to cause cancer in mice when given in large doses. Saffrole is not soluble in water and is not present in significant quantities in traditional teas. However, the U.S. Food and Drug Administration banned the interstate marketing of sassafras for sassafras tea in 1976 because of its saffrole content.

☞ DIRECTIONS: Place 1 ounce of sassafras root bark in 1 quart of water. Cover, bring to a boil, and simmer on the lowest heat for fifteen minutes. Let the water cool to room temperature. Strain and drink 1 cup a day for seven to fourteen days.

SARSAPARILLA: Sarsaparilla *(Smilax officinalis)*, which grows mainly in the semi-tropical areas of North America, was one of the most important "new" plants discovered in the colonies by the Europeans, and it was shipped in large amounts back to Europe as a blood purifier and treatment for syphilis. It is still used today as a blood purifier in the folk medicine of Pennsylvania Germans and throughout Appalachia. In some parts of the mountains, it is considered a second-best substitute for the more potent sassafras. The German government has judged that no scientific evidence exists to support the use of sarsaparilla for any medical condition. Use for longer than seven to fourteen days is not recommended.

☞ DIRECTIONS: Simmer 1 ounce of dried and chopped sarsaparilla root in 1 quart of water for twenty to thirty minutes. Strain and drink 1 or 2 cups a day for up to seven days.

YERBA MANSA: In Beatrice Roeder's *Chicano Folk Medicine from Los Angeles,* folk scholar Laura Curtin, as expert on Southwestern traditional medicine, states: "No other plant enjoys so wide a medicinal fame or has a higher repute," than yerba mansa *(Anemopsis californica)*. Spanish settlers learned the plant's uses from the Maricopa, Pima, and Tewa Indian groups. "Yerba mansa" is short for "yerba del indio manso," or "herb of the tamed Indians." American physicians of the Eclectic school (see sidebar, "Eclectic Medicine," page 25) began using it in 1877, and continued to do so until the 1940s. These physicians recommended the plant as a remedy for treating conditions of the mucous membranes—conditions that involved a stuffy sensation in the head and throat, a cough with expectoration, or mucous discharges from the bowels or urinary tract.

☞ DIRECTIONS: Place 1 ounce of yerba mansa in 1 quart of water, bring to a boil, and simmer for twenty to thirty minutes. Let stand until cool. Drink 1 to 3 cups each day for a week or two.

GREENS: Pennsylvania Germans make a ritual of "thinning the blood" in the spring by eating "blutreinigungsmittel," which includes such greens as dandelion *(Taraxacum officinale)* and plantain *(Plantago major)*. Farmers in Indiana purify the blood by consuming the greens of the two plants lamb's quarters *(Chenopodium album)* and wild mustard *(Brassica kaber)*.

☞ DIRECTIONS: Be sure to collect the greens in areas that have not been sprayed with pesticides! Eat them raw in salads or stir fry them with a little olive oil, garlic, and lemon. Eat as often as desired.

✿ Boils and ✿
Carbuncles

▦ ▦ ▦

Boils—furuncles is the medical term—are tender, inflamed swellings centered around hair follicles in the scalp or skin. They result from infection by various strains of *Staphylococcus* bacteria. Carbuncles are clusters of boils, often appearing on the nape of the neck. Boils and carbuncles may appear on otherwise healthy individuals, although diabetes mellitus, debilitating diseases, and old age may predispose a person to the condition. Boils do not normally present a health hazard, but carbuncles may be accompanied by fever and exhaustion. Boils on the nose or in the central area of the face require medical attention and treatment with antibiotics, however, because the bacterial infection can spread easily from that area to the brain.

Conventional and traditional treatment for simple boils is identical: Applications of moist heat until the boil comes to a head and drains spontaneously. Surgical incision or squeezing can spread the infection internally and should be avoided. For more serious infections, the conventional treatment is antibiotic therapy. Besides the use of poultices and disinfectant washes, traditional medicine also centers on purifying the blood through building up the strength of the immune system to resist bacterial infection.

Remedies

CHAMOMILE POULTICE: The folk medicine of the American Southwest recommends a poultice of hot chamomile tea *(Matricaria recutita)* for treating boils. Chamomile contains essential oils that have antiseptic, antibacterial, and anti-inflammatory properties.

☞ DIRECTIONS: Place ½ ounce of chamomile flowers in a 1-pint canning jar and cover with boiling water. Cover the jar tightly and let stand for fifteen minutes. Strain the liquid and apply the hot mash directly to the boil. Cover with a cloth, and keep the cloth moist with the strained liquid. Do this remedy every two to three hours for twenty minutes at a time, until the boil comes to a head and drains.

CORNMEAL POULTICE: A folk remedy of the Aztecs—which survives today in the folk medicine of the American Southwest—was to apply a poultice of cornmeal and hot water to the boil. The same method was used by the Cherokee Indians, who passed the remedy along to the Appalachians. The remedy is still used today in rural Indiana. It is the texture of the corn and its ability to hold the heat of water—not the medicinal properties of the corn—that are responsible for the value of this treatment.

☞ DIRECTIONS: In a pot, bring ½ cup of water to a boil. Turn off the heat and add cornmeal to make a thick paste. Apply the mixture to the boil, and cover with a cloth. Repeat every one to two hours until the boil comes to a head and drains.

ONION POULTICE: Onion *(Allium cepa)* poultices were used among eastern American Indian tribes, European colonists of the eastern states, Appalachian folk healers, and contemporary Indiana farmers and Hispanic New Mexicans to treat boils. Onions contain antiseptic chemicals and irritating constituents that draw blood and heat to the affected area.

☞ DIRECTIONS: Place a thick slice of onion over

the boil and keep in place by wrapping with a cloth. Change every three to four hours until the boil comes to a head and drains.

EGG SKIN POULTICE: A 19th century remedy for treating boils in the eastern United States was to apply the soft outer skin of a hard-boiled egg directly to the boil. It is now a commonly used remedy in contemporary New England, Appalachia, and southwestern Colorado.

☞ DIRECTIONS: Hard boil an egg. Crack off the shell and carefully peel the outer skin off the egg. Wet it and apply the egg skin directly to the boil and cover with a clean cloth.

PORK POULTICE: Salt pork or bacon poultices are commonly used to treat various skin afflictions throughout New England and Appalachia. To treat a boil, you can try using a pork poultice. The poultice does not need to be hot, but the meat used should be fat meat. It is probably the constituents in the fat and the salt used to preserve the meat that bring the boil to a head.

☞ DIRECTIONS: Roll some fatty pork or bacon in salt and place the meat between two pieces of cloth. Apply the poultice to the boil. Repeat throughout the day until the boil comes to a head and drains.

BREAD AND MILK POULTICE: Poultices made of bread and milk have been used to treat boils in New England, Appalachia, Indiana, and among Hispanics in southwestern Colorado. It is the drawing nature of the mixture and the heat of the poultice that make this remedy work.

☞ DIRECTIONS: Heat 1 cup of milk and add 3 teaspoons of salt. (Add the salt slowly so it will not curdle the milk.) Simmer the mixture for ten minutes. Thicken the mixture by adding flour or crumbled bread pieces. Divide the mixture into four poultices and apply one poultice to the boil every half hour. The poultice may also be applied before bedtime, held in place with a cloth, and kept on overnight.

NUTMEG: A popular remedy for treating boils in New England, Appalachia, and parts of the American Southwest is eating nutmeg (*Myristica fragrans*). Nutmeg is also sometimes applied directly

A Gypsy Formula

A gypsy formula from Spain for treating boils combines several of the remedies already described: Make a tea of burdock and stinging nettle leaves and add 2 crushed garlic cloves. Drink a cup three times a day on an empty stomach, before meals. This tea from across the Atlantic is remarkably similar to one used in the contemporary herbalism of the Pacific Northwest that uses burdock and nettle without the garlic.

to the boil as a poultice. Nutmeg stim-ulates the body's circulation, which conceivably could assist the body in fighting the infection of the boil.

☞ DIRECTIONS: Grind nutmeg. Stir ½ teaspoon into a cup of hot water and drink. Do this three to four times a day for up to three days.

Burns and Sunburns

❊ ❊ ❊

Burns are medically classified in two ways: by the depth of the burn and by the amount of body area the burn covers. Deep burns and burns covering large surface areas require medical examination. The most superficial burn is the first-degree burn, which is typical of a simple sunburn. A second-degree burn penetrates deeper into the skin and is usually accompanied by blisters. Third-degree burns involve deep tissue destruction. Third-degree burns may not blister, so they at first may appear to be less serious than they are. Often the skin looks whitish or charred. The chief risk of second- and third-degree burns is infection, and the more surface area that is affected, the more serious the risk.

Infection may enter through ruptured blisters or through seemingly intact skin that has been burned. Folk remedies are inappropriate for these burns, and some could actually promote infection. Conventional treatment for simple superficial burns includes cooling the tissues as soon as possible to reduce inflammation and blistering, and applying soothing ointments. This is the same strategy used by folk healers throughout the world. Some of the folk remedies below, such as aloe vera, are disinfectants and probably helped to save lives endangered by infected burns in the past.

Remedies

BUTTER AND CREAM: A kitchen burn remedy that

comes in handy in most houses is butter, which is mentioned in the folk literature of New England, North Carolina, Northern Georgia, Indiana, and the San Luis Valley of Colorado. Butterfat contains fats that have antimicrobial properties. Thus, butter may help disinfect as well as soothe a burn. An alternative to butter, in the folklore of the Amish dairy farmers, is to dip the burned area in cream.

☞ DIRECTIONS: After dipping a minor burn in cold water and drying it, apply butter or cream.

BAKING SODA POULTICE: Baking soda, sometimes used in combination with other substances, is mentioned as a burn remedy in folk remedy sources from New England and Indiana and among the Seventh Day Adventists.

☞ DIRECTIONS: To treat a minor burn, mix baking soda and enough raw egg whites to form a paste. Place the mash directly on the burn and cover with gauze.

BAKING SODA BATH: The Seventh Day Adventists recommend a baking soda bath for treating sunburn.

☞ DIRECTIONS: Fill a tub with 94–98°F water. Add a cup of commercial baking soda. Soak in the tub for thirty to sixty

Everything Oily

Conventional treatment for a minor burn is to first dip the burned area in cold water, dry it, and then cover the area with an oily salve or ointment. Oily substances used in the folk medicines of various cultures have included, besides butter: egg yolks, lard, olive oil, bear fat, chicken fat, goose "grease," skunk oil, mutton tallow, deer tallow, cocoa butter, petroleum jelly, fish oil, axle grease, and, believe it or not, kerosene.

Fire Doctors and Special Prayers

In Appalachian and southern culture, it is believed by some that certain individuals—called "fire doctors"—have the ability to "talk" fire out of a burn. The belief is so strong that some individuals with serious burns will refuse any other medical treatment. In Louisiana folk medicine, the "fire passages" of the Bible are recited by the fire doctor. The identity of the passages is closely guarded and passed on from one healer to another only at the time of a fire doctor's death. In The Frank C. Brown Collection of North Carolina Folklore, one prayer recited by a northern Georgia fire doctor is: "The mother of God went over the fiery fields. She had in her hand a fiery brand. The fire did not go out; it did not go in. In the name of the Father, the Son, and the Holy Ghost. Amen." The prayer is repeated three times; the fire doctor blows on the burn and wets the area each time.

minutes. Let the skin dry naturally, without using a towel.

VINEGAR: Vinegar washes are recommended in folk remedies from New England and New Mexico. Vinegar is both astringent and antiseptic, and, like cool water, it helps to prevent blisters.

☞ DIRECTIONS: Apply vinegar to the burn every few minutes. Dilute the vinegar if the skin is very sensitive.

ALOE VERA: The juice of the aloe vera plant has been used as a burn remedy by practically every culture. Aloe vera is recommended as a burn remedy—for sunburn to serious third-degree burns—in the folk literature of American Indians, New Englanders, the Amish, Indiana residents, Gypsies, residents of northern Georgia, and Chinese immigrants. Aloe also acts as a disinfectant and reduces bacteria in burns.

Physiomedicalist Medicine

The most influential folk herbalist in United States history is Samuel Thomson (1769–1843), a self-educated "doctor" from New Hampshire. Thomson advocated the use of simple herbal remedies and severely criticized the methods of the medical doctors of the day. By the 1840s, his "Thomsonian" movement had claimed as many as a million adherents—about 20 percent of the American population at the time—who purchased his books of home remedies or ordered his herbal remedies through the mail. Emerging from this folk movement around 1840 came the Physiomedicalist school of medicine, which included doctors who used Thomson's philosophy and methods. Physiomedicalist medicine in the United States passed away with the death of its most prominent adherent, William Cook, M.D., in 1899. However, an English doctor named A.I. Coffin, who had studied with Thomson in the 1820s, and also with American Indian doctors, had spread the movement to England. He lectured in small towns across that country, and the resulting folk movement that sprang up there was similar to the Thomsonian herbalism of the United States. Physiomedicalism profoundly influenced British herbalism from that time on. Today, herbalists are licensed in England, and their training and approach remain strongly influenced by Physiomedicalism.

☞ DIRECTIONS: For a small burn, break off a leaf, slice it down the middle, and rub the gel on the skin. To make a poultice of aloe, place the cut leaf on the burned area, and wrap the area with gauze. You can also apply store-bought aloe gel or juice. An alternate formula is to extend the aloe vera sap with olive oil. Here's how: Add 8 ounces of extra virgin olive oil to 2 ounces of fresh squeezed aloe vera sap. (Place the sap in a large bowl and add the oil a few drops at a time while stirring.) Apply directly to the burn area.

PLANTAIN: Plantain (*Plantago major*), a popular remedy for wounds, bites, and stings, is also recommended for treating burns in the folk literature of the Seneca Indians. Contemporary New Englanders and Hispanics of the American Southwest also encourage its use. The plantain leaf contains at least 15 constituents with identified anti-inflammatory properties, 17 constituents with bactericidal properties, 6 analgesics, and 5 antiseptics. It also contains the constituent allantoin, which promotes cell proliferation and tissue healing.

☞ DIRECTIONS: Crush some fresh plantain leaves and rub the juice directly onto the burn area.

TOBACCO: An American Indian treatment for burns is to wash the area in tobacco tea. Indiana medical folklore suggests applying a wad of chewing tobacco to the burned area.

☞ DIRECTIONS: Remove the tobacco from a package of cigarettes and add it to 1 quart of water. Boil the water until the volume is reduced to 1 pint. Strain and let cool to room temperature. Wash the burn area with the tea as often as you'd like.

POTATO POULTICE: Some residents of New England, Indiana, and North Carolina have reported using potato poultices in treating burns. The same use is widespread in the folk medicine of India and has even attracted the attention of researchers there. Potato poultices were tested on severe burns in a 1990 clinical trial at a children's hospital in Bombay, India. A control group received a conventional treatment with an ointment of silver sulfadiazine. The test group also received the sulfadiazine, in addition to a dressing of potato peels. The patients in the latter group showed faster healing than the control patients. Potato treatments without the conventional antibiotic ointment may promote infection on the open wounds of severe burns, however. (A 1996 trial at a burn unit in Maharashtra, India, compared the efficacy of potato treatments to honey-impregnated gauze. The honey treatments were more effective and prevented infection, whereas the patients receiving potato poultices showed persistent infections in their burns within the first week of the trial.)

☞ DIRECTIONS: Apply a poultice of grated raw potato directly to the burn and hold it in place with a cloth. Change the poultice every one to two hours until the burn heals. This treatment is not appropriate for burns with broken skin or ruptured blisters.

Manure R_x

One remedy, though perhaps unappealing and unsanitary, is to apply manure or excrement to a burn. Although the texture of manure may be soothing to the burn, if there is any break in the skin, the risk of infection is very high. In *Country Folk Remedies: Tales of Skunk Oil, Sassafras Tea and Other Old-Time Remedies Gathered by Elisabeth Janos*, New England folklorist Elizabeth Janos relates one folk narrative: "I took about two cups of chicken manure and the same amount of pure lard. I boiled them together for about fifteen minutes, then let it cool. It makes a somewhat smelly yellow salve. I used it on him three to four times a day. In about two weeks he was healed, and no scar was left." Cow manure is used by other New Englanders, and dog excrement is used by Mexican Indians.

HONEY: Honey is a universal folk remedy to disinfect wounds and burns throughout the world. It is highly regarded in the folk literature of the Amish, Chinese immigrants, Indiana residents, and residents of the American Southwest. Honey naturally attracts water, and, when applied to a burn or wound, draws fluids out of the tissues, effectively cleaning the wound. Furthermore, most bacteria cannot live in the presence of honey. Honey is sometimes applied to gauze and used to dress severe burns in conventional medicine. In the early 1990s, physicians at a hospital in Maharashtra, India, performed clinical trials comparing honey-impregnated gauze with three different conventional burn treatments, and the honey treatment was superior in each case.

In a 1991 study, the doctors compared the honey-gauze to gauze treated with silver sulfadiazine. In 52 patients treated with honey, 91 percent of wounds were sterile within seven days. In the 52 patients treated with silver sulfadiazine, 93 percent of wounds still showed signs of infection after seven days. The burns of the honey-treated patients began to heal in seven days, while, for the other group, healing began on average in 13 days. Of the wounds treated with honey, 87 percent healed within 15 days; only 10 percent of the wounds healed in the control group during that time. Important: The honey also provided greater pain relief and resulted in less scarring.

☞ DIRECTIONS: Apply honey to a piece of sterile gauze, and place directly on the burn, honey side to the skin. Change the dressing three to four times a day. Be sure to seek medical attention for serious burns.

❦ Cold and Flu ❦

▧ ▧ ▧

A simple common cold is a collection of familiar symptoms signaling an infection of the upper respiratory tract, which includes the nose, throat, and sinuses. At least five major categories of viruses cause colds. One of these groups, and perhaps the most common, the rhinoviruses, includes a minimum of 100 different viruses. The viruses that cause a cold reproduce in the mucous membranes. The viruses do not penetrate deeper into the body—into the gastrointestinal tract, for example—because they cannot survive at the higher body temperatures there.

Although we often say "colds and flu" in the same breath, influenza is a very different disease from the common cold. The influenza virus takes up residence mainly in the throat and bronchial tract. If you have the flu, you usually have a fever, and a fever is not usually present in a cold. The fever usually passes within three days, but the fatigue, muscle aches, and cough that result from the flu can linger for weeks. Influenza will not seriously injure a normally healthy person, but those with preexisting lung conditions, the elderly, and others with weakened resistance are especially prone to the flu's deadly effects.

Flu is known as the "Last of the Great Plagues" because it kills so many people worldwide each year, including about 20,000 Americans. And when highly virulent flu strains periodically erupt, the death toll can rise even higher. For example, a flu epidemic just after World War I killed more than 30 million people worldwide.

The conventional treatment for flu in those at high risk for fatal complications is immunization in late fall with a flu vaccine. Immunization is also recommended for those who care for such high-risk patients. The antiviral drug ribavarin can be taken as well; it may be effective in preventing severe pneumonia caused by the influenza virus.

Some patients request antibiotics from their doctors to treat a cold or flu episode, and, unfortunately, many doctors comply. Antibiotic drugs are good only for bacterial infections and are ineffective against colds and flu. In fact, taking them inappropriately may promote the development of drug-resistant bacterial strains and may render the antibiotics ineffective later on when the patient really needs them. The drug resistant strains can also be passed on to others.

Aspirin and other pain-killing drugs are also inappropriate treatments for cold and flu. Even though they may provide some temporary relief, they may suppress the immune system and can actually prolong the infection. And giving aspirin to children for colds and flu is a no-no. In rare cases, it can lead to the development of Reye syndrome, a serious and often fatal neurological disorder.

Remedies

ECHINACEA: Echinacea (*Echinacea angustifolia, Echinacea purpurea*) is, without a doubt, the most commonly used folk remedy for treating colds and flu in the United States today. In fact, echinacea is the best-selling medicinal herb in the country.

Echinacea was used as a remedy by the American Indians of the Great Plains states. The tribes residing in those areas used the herb for all manner of infectious diseases. Eclectic physicians, a now-defunct North American school of doctors who used herbs as medicines, adopted the use of echinacea in the mid-1880s. By 1920, it was the remedy they prescribed the most. The use of echinacea spread to Germany in the 1930s, where it remains an approved medicine today—used to treat colds, flu, and other conditions related to underlying deficiencies of the immune system.

Echinacea is also famous in the contemporary medical herbalism of Britain, Australia, and North America for its ability to "abort" a cold or flu. German clinical trials show that echinacea, taken preventively during cold and flu season, can reduce the frequency and severity of a viral infection. In fact, if echinacea is taken at the first onset of symptoms, the cold may never develop at all. Once a cold has set in, however, the other remedies in the section may be more beneficial.

☞ DIRECTIONS: Purchase a tincture of echinacea at a health food store, herb shop, or drugstore. At the first sign of a cold or flu, take 1 teaspoon of the tincture every hour for three hours. If the infection persists, take 1 dropperful of the tincture every three hours.

ELDER FLOWERS: Elderberry comprises about 13 species of deciduous shrubs native to North America and Europe. European settlers brought elderberry plants with them to the American colonies. The Paiute and Shoshone Indians in the Rocky Mountain region used the leaves and flowers of a North American species of elderberry to treat colds, flu, and fevers.

A tea made of elderberry flowers is approved by the German government as a medicine for colds, especially if a cough is present. The flower tea is also used to treat colds and flu in the folk medicine of contemporary Indiana. The Michigan Amish use the tea as well.

Recent research in Israel and Panama has shown that elderberry juice stimulates the immune system and also directly inhibits the influenza virus. Con-

Sniffing Tea

Folk traditions frequently advise a cold or flu victim to sip hot fragrant teas. Most of the herbs in this section contain aromatic oils that have antibacterial, antiviral, antifungal, and anti-inflammatory actions. The oils escape with the steam of hot tea. (The steam also releases the oils' fragrance.) The steam delivers the oil's constituents directly to the surface of the mucous membranes, where they attack the invading organism causing the cold. Elder, ginger, yarrow, mint, thyme, horsemint, beebalm, lemon balm, catnip, garlic, onions, and mustard are all herbs that contain such aromatic oils.

stituents in the plant's flowers and berries seem to have immunosuppressant properties that help inactivate the influenza virus, halting its spread. Elderberry has been shown to be effective against eight different strains of the flu virus. Drinking too much elderberry tea, more than indicated in the directions below, however, can leave you feeling nauseous. And, because of a documented diuretic effect, prolonged use may result in hypokalemia, or potassium loss. Avoid the use of elder during pregnancy and lactation.

☞ DIRECTIONS: Place ½ ounce of elderberry flowers in a 1-quart canning jar and fill with boiling water. Cover and let steep for twenty minutes. Strain and pour a cup of the tea. Sweeten with honey. Take 1 cup once every four hours when you have a cold or flu. Wrap yourself up in warm blankets after drinking the tea to help induce sweating.

BONESET: The herb boneset (*Eupatorium perfoliatum*) got its name during an influenza epidemic in Pennsylvania in the 1700s. The flu was called "breakbone fever"; the word *breakbone* referred to the muscle aches and pains that accompanied the virus. Taking the herb, however, proved to "set the bones" and relieve the aches. The colonists learned the use of the plant from the Cherokee and Iroquois Indians and other eastern American Indian tribes.

The use of boneset for treating colds and flu spread to Europe. Today, some German medical schools continue to study its use. Boneset is frequently prescribed in Germany for treating acute viral infections, for which antibiotic drugs are not effective. The herb also continues to be used today in the folk medicine of Indiana and southern Illinois.

Constituents have been identified in boneset that

Sweating It Out

Sweating is essential to cooling the body during a fever. Many traditional folk remedies use herbs for this purpose. These diaphoretic herbs have constituents that, when eaten, increase the blood circulation to the skin, which causes perspiration and ultimately lowers the fever.

It is essential to drink plenty of fluids when taking these herbs, however, or dehydration may result. Elder, ginger, yarrow, mint, boneset, pennyroyal, thyme, horsemint, beebalm, lemon balm, catnip, and garlic are all diaphoretic herbs. They're most effective when taken as hot teas. After drinking the tea, go to bed, wrap up in warm blankets, and sweat it out. Continue to drink plenty of fluids.

are both immune-stimulating and anti-inflammatory. Do not overdo it with boneset, however, because it can induce vomiting if taken in large quantities. It was actually used for that purpose in the 18th and 19th centuries. Boneset is also know to have constituents that are allergenic. Boneset should be avoided during pregnancy and lactation.

☞ DIRECTIONS: Place 1 teaspoon of dried boneset leaves in a cup and fill with boiling water. Let steep for fifteen minutes. Strain and drink the tea while it's warm. Go to bed immediately, wrapping yourself in blankets. Don't drink more than 1 cup every four hours and no more than 3 cups a day. Stop taking boneset if you begin to feel nauseous.

YARROW: The ancient Greeks used yarrow (*Achillea millefolium*) as a remedy for colds, flu, and fever. At least 18 American Indian tribes from all corners of North America used yarrow for the same purpose. The early colonists throughout North America used yarrow as a household medicine for a wide variety of ailments, usually conditions that were infectious or inflammatory in nature. The use of yarrow tea for colds and flu survives today in the folk medicine of North Carolina, Indiana, and upstate New York. Yarrow has documented anti-inflammatory, antispasmodic, diuretic, mild sedative, and moderate antibacterial activities.

☞ DIRECTIONS: Place 1 ounce of dried or fresh yarrow in a 1-quart canning jar. Fill the jar with boiling water and cover tightly. Let steep for twenty minutes. Strain and pour a cup and sweeten with honey. Take 2 or 3 cups a day, bundling up in blankets and resting in bed after each cup.

GINGER: Ginger tea is a cold remedy mentioned in the folk literature of New England, Appalachia, North Carolina, Indiana, and even China. Ginger induces sweating, which helps to cool the body during fever. Ginger contains 12 different aromatic anti-inflammatory compounds, including some with aspirinlike effects. Its other proven actions result from its antinauseant and antivertigo properties.

Ginger also has carminative (gas relieving), diaphoretic (sweat inducing), and antispasmodic activities.

☞ DIRECTIONS: Cut a fresh ginger root (about the size of your thumb) into thin slices. Place the slices in 1 quart of water. Bring to a boil. Cover the pot and simmer on the lowest possible heat for thirty minutes. Let cool for thirty minutes more. Strain and drink ½ to 1 cup three to five times a day. Sweeten with honey, as desired.

PEPPERMINT: Peppermint (*Mentha piperita*) is a folk remedy used in Indiana to treat colds. Cornmint (*Mentha arvensis*), a close relative of the plant, is used in China for the same purpose. Both plants, when taken as a hot tea, induce sweating and help to cool a fever. Also, the essential oils in the plants, including menthol, act as

Starve a Cold?

"Starve a fever, feed a cold" is an aphorism of folk wisdom—one that you should try not to get confused. If you feed a fever or starve a cold, you may be making your fever worse and actually prolonging it.

During a fever, the body's metabolism goes into overdrive to produce white blood cells and antibodies to fight the infection. If you fast, your body doesn't have to produce digestive enzymes, freeing up the system to make more immune system components.

For a usually healthy person, fasting for 24 hours increases the activity of white blood cells by about 20 percent. So, at the first sign of fever, fast on liquids, carefully avoiding sugary juices, until your temperature returns to normal. And don't worry about starving—the body holds plenty of nutrients in reserve.

decongestants when drunk as a tea or inhaled. Peppermint also has antispasmodic and carminative properties.

☞ DIRECTIONS: Place ½ ounce of peppermint leaves in a 1-quart jar. Fill the jar with boiling water and cover tightly. Let steep twenty minutes. Strain the liquid and drink 2 or 3 cups a day. Wrap yourself in blankets and rest in bed after each cup.

THYME: Thyme tea (*Thymus vulgaris*) is recommended as a treatment for cold or flu in the folk medicine of Indiana and China. Thyme taken in the form of a hot tea also induces sweating and helps to cool a fever. In addition, its constituent oil, thymol, is a powerful expectorant and antiseptic. The constituent readily disperses in the steam of a hot tea. Inhaling the steam may effectively spread the thymol throughout the mucous membranes of the upper respiratory tract and bronchial tree. Thus, thymol may help inhibit

bacteria, viruses, or fungi from infecting the membranes. Thyme also has mild analgesic and antipyretic (fever reducing) properties.

This remedy from Indiana suggests sipping the tea slowly while inhaling its fragrance. In China, the same method is used as a preventive— for when colds or flu are "going around."

☞ DIRECTIONS: Put 1 teaspoon of dried thyme leaves in a cup and fill with boiling water. Let steep for five minutes while inhaling the fumes through both the nose and mouth. Then, strain the tea, sweeten with honey, and sip slowly. Go to bed and bundle up warmly in blankets.

HORSEMINT AND BEEBALM: Two closely related species, horsemint (*Monarda punctata*) and beebalm (*Monarda menthaefolia, M. didyma*), are used in folk medicine similarly to the way thyme is used. (Horsemint is native to the eastern United States; beebalm to the Rocky Mountains.) Both plants, like thyme, contain high amounts of the constituent thymol, which acts as an expectorant and antiseptic (see "Thyme," page 111). Both plants also induce sweating and can help cool a fever.

☞ DIRECTIONS: Put 1 teaspoon of dried leaves of either plant in a cup and fill with boiling water. Let steep for five minutes while inhaling the fumes through both the nose and mouth. Strain, sweeten with honey, and sip the tea slowly. Do this three to five times a day.

LEMON BALM: Several Indiana residents responding to a poll of folk remedies in the 1980s recommended lemon balm (*Melissa officinalis*) tea for cold and flu. The plant, which is native to southern Europe and northern Africa, now grows throughout North America as well. Lemon balm has long been used as a relaxing and sweat-inducing herb. The 12th century German mystic and healer Hildegarde von Bingen stated, "Lemon balm contains within it the virtues of a dozen other plants."

Lemon balm is approved today by the German government as a medicine for digestive complaints and sleeping disorders, though it is not recommended specifically for colds or flu. Its aromatic oils contain antiviral compounds that may help disinfect the mucous membranes, however. Of the sweat-inducing herbs included in this section, lemon balm is probably the mildest and the most suitable for use in children. Lemon balm is also a mild sedative and can help relax a restless patient suffering from cold or flu.

☞ DIRECTIONS: Place 1 teaspoon of the dried herb in a cup and fill with boiling water. Let steep for ten minutes. Inhale the steam from the cup. Strain and drink up to 4 cups a day. Sweeten with honey as desired.

GARLIC: The recommendation to take garlic for

colds comes from New England, the American Southwest, and all the way from China. Garlic has been used for colds, bronchial problems, and fevers in cultures throughout the world since the dawn of written medical history—even the ancient Egyptians used it to treat cough and fever.

Garlic's constituents are antibacterial, antiviral, and antifungal. Garlic also stimulates the immune system, increasing the body's resistance to invaders. In addition, garlic is an expectorant and induces sweating, helping to reduce fever. Garlic has been approved as a medicine for colds and coughs and a variety of other illnesses by the pharmaceutical regulatory commission of the European Union, a confederation of modern European nations that has dropped trade barriers and is working toward economic regulation and a common currency. Garlic can also lower cholesterol and thin the blood. Note that garlic taken in high doses can irritate the stomach.

☞ DIRECTIONS: Blend 3 cloves of garlic in a blender with a little water. (A clove must be cut or crushed to release its constituents.) If you want, add half a lemon, skin and all, to the garlic. Put the contents in a cup and fill the cup with boiling water. Let steep for five minutes, inhaling the fragrance. Strain, add honey, and drink the entire cup in sips. Do this two to three times a day while you have a cold or flu or once a day to prevent infection during epidemics.

Alternately, peel and chop 3 whole garlic bulbs and soak them in 1 pint of wine (red or white) in a closed container for a month. Shake the jar once a day. Then, strain and take 1 tablespoon of the wine each day as a preventive measure.

ONIONS: Onions are used to treat colds in virtually every folk tradition in North America—whether eaten raw, roasted, or boiled; taken in the form of teas, milk, or wine; worn in a sock or in a bag around the neck; or applied to the chest as a poultice. Wild onions have been used for the same purpose by American Indian tribes in every region of the country. Using onions to treat colds continues today in the folk medicine of New England, upstate New York, North Carolina, Appalachia, Indiana, and within Chinese cultures throughout North America.

The constituents in onions—the same that cause onion's volatile vapors to burn the eyes—are antimicrobial. Onions also have expectorant qualities, which induce the flow of healthy cleansing mucus. Onions induce sweating as well, helping to cool a fever.

☞ DIRECTIONS: Cut up 1 whole large onion and simmer in a covered pot for twenty minutes. Strain if desired to remove pulp. Drink a cup of the tea three to four times daily when you have a cold or flu.

Alternately, try chewing raw onions—but don't swallow until the onions are thoroughly chewed. Note: Chewing too many onions can cause stomach irritation.

To make an onion poultice for chest colds, slice 3 large onions, discarding the outer paper-like skin. Cover with water and simmer for twenty minutes. Strain. Layer the cooked onions between two cloths. Apply to the chest for twenty to thirty minutes.

LEMON: The contemporary folk traditions of New England and Indiana call for drinking "hot lemonade" during a cold or flu. The

Hot Water Treatments

Treatments for colds and flu often emphasize using hot water for hot steam baths, gargles, and nasal irrigations. These remedies are mentioned in the folk literature of 19th century German immigrants as well as present-day Seventh Day Adventists. Such water methods have a sound basis in microbiology: The viruses that infect the mucous membranes cannot survive even at normal body temperatures. Thus, by washing the membranes with water even hotter than the body's core temperature, or flooding the membranes with steam, infecting viruses are killed.

practice is at least as old as the ancient Romans.

Lemon juice, like vinegar, is acidic. Drinking it helps to acidify the mucous membranes, making the membranes inhospitable to bacteria or viruses. Lemon oil, which gives the juice its fragrance, is like a pharmacy in itself—it contains antibacterial, antiviral, antifungal, and anti-inflammatory constituents. Five of the constituents are specifically active against the influenza virus. Lemon oil is also an expectorant. And lemon is very tasty—its flavor is used to promote compli-ance in taking cold and flu products.

☞ DIRECTIONS: Place 1 chopped whole lemon—skin, pulp, and all—in a pot and add 1 cup of boiling water. While letting the mixture steep for five minutes, inhale the fumes. Then, strain and drink. Do this at the onset of a cold, and repeat three to four times a day for the duration of the cold.

VINEGAR: A cold remedy from Indiana calls for inhaling the fumes of vinegar. This remedy is as old as ancient Greece—
continued on page 117

Weather and Illness

⊞ ⊞ ⊞

Bad weather and bad health are often believed to be related. Many people believe that certain physical changes or plain ol' aches and pains—such as arthritis in the joints—can predict changes in the weather. And frequent or severe changes in the weather are believed to actually cause some people to get sick.

One common belief in North America is that a warm winter is likely to result in an increase in disease in the spring and summer. Settlers in the upper Midwest noticed this phenomenon over a century ago. Warm winters were usually followed by epidemics of fevers that were associated with swampy environments. A similar belief is that winters with repeated freezing and thawing make some people more susceptible to disease.

Sunstroke is a very real risk in many areas of the country, especially for those individuals who work outdoors. Some people believe that you can avoid getting sunstroke by carrying charms, such as elder leaves or the rattle from a rattlesnake, in your clothes.

Wind and night air can also be seen as dangerous, especially to children. Children, particularly babies, may be considered to be unusually susceptible to catching colds and other ailments. New parents are often cautioned not to take a young child out at night because the night air is bad for the infant. Colic is sometimes said to have been caused by taking a child out on a windy day. Some Pennsylvania Germans think that children are more likely to get sick in the spring. They believe that the March winds bring diseases that children are very likely to catch. Another belief is that sleeping with the east wind blowing on you will cause you to go insane!

the Greek physician Hippocrates recommended the treatment for coughs and respiratory infections. Vinegar is a weak acid. Inhaling its fumes changes the acidity of the mucous membranes in the upper respiratory tract, making the membranes inhospitable to viruses. Due to its acidic nature, avoid splashing vinegar into the eyes or onto cuts.

☞ DIRECTIONS: In a jar, pour ½ cup of boiling water over ½ cup of vinegar. Gently inhale the steam. Be careful not to burn yourself.

MUSTARD PLASTER: The mustard plaster has been used medicinally in Europe at least since the time of the ancient Romans. The contemporary Amish still recommend it for treating chest colds and bronchitis. It works mainly by increasing circulation, perspiration, and heat in the afflicted area. In addition, when its irritant antimicrobial and anti-inflammatory volatile substances are inhaled, mustard may also have a medicinal effect on the mucous membranes of the upper respiratory tract. The active principle is allylisothiocyanate, which is also present in horseradish and watercress.

☞ DIRECTIONS: Mix ½ cup mustard with 1 cup flour. Stir warm water into the mustard and flour mixture until a paste is formed. This allows for the active principle to be released. Spread the mixture on a piece of cotton or muslin that has been soaked in hot water. Cover with a second piece of dry material. Lay the moist side of the poultice across the person's chest or back. Leave the poultice on for fifteen to thirty minutes. Remove promptly if the person experiences any discomfort. (Be careful not to blister or burn the skin. You may want to lift the cloth every five minutes or so to check how red the skin is.)

VAPORIZE IT: The contemporary Amish suggest using a vaporizer and adding essential oils to the water, such as pine, cedar, or mint. Many of the aromatic constituents of these plants have antimicrobial properties. If you can smell the aroma, then at least a small amount of the constituent has reached your mucous membranes and may assist in killing viruses there. Peppermint oil also contains menthol, which acts as a deconges-

tant. Excessive inhalation can be hazardous to sensitive or allergic young children, however.

☞ DIRECTIONS: Add a few drops of essential oils to the water of a commercial vaporizer. If you've purchased concentrated essential oils, be sure to dilute them with at least five parts of a carrier oil (such as almond oil) before adding them to the water.

Beware of Alcohol

Several folk traditions from the eastern United States suggest taking alcohol to treat a cold. In fact, a recommendation from a collection of Indiana folklore suggests hanging your hat on a bed post and drinking whiskey until you see two hats!

Getting drunk may well help you to forget the misery of a cold, but, from a medical standpoint, it is not such a good idea. Drinking to the point of intoxication depresses the immune system. Alcohol reduces the rate at which white blood cells engulf invading organisms; it also depresses antibody production. Thus, the duration and severity of a cold can only be made worse by alcohol consumption during the infection. Alcohol can also make your cold worse if you are exposed to cold air. The alcohol dilates the blood vessels near the surface of the skin, which promotes loss of body heat. The body then has to work even harder to maintain its normal temperature or a healthy fever.

Place the vaporizer next to the sick bed and keep it running around the clock.

SALT WATER: According to New England and Indiana folk medicine, a good remedy for treating a head cold is sniffing warm salt water. The salt itself is antimicrobial, and the heat from the warm water kills the viruses that attack the mucous membranes (see sidebar, "Hot Water Treatments," page 115).

☞ DIRECTIONS: Put ¼ teaspoon of salt in a glass of hot or warm water. Sniff some of the water. Do this after being exposed to someone with a cold or flu or at the first sign of infec-tion. Repeat every three to four hours while suffering from a cold.

WATER TREATMENTS: The Seventh Day Adventists suggest a variety of water treatments for curing a cold.

☞ DIRECTIONS: At the first sign of a cold, put your feet in hot water. Keep the water hot for twenty minutes. Then run cold water over your feet and dry them. Cover your feet well or wrap yourself in a blanket and go to bed for half an hour.

Also, you can try drawing hot water up into the nasal passages and then blowing the water back out. Just

Chicken Soup

Chicken soup is a universal remedy for colds. It is mentioned in the folk literature of New England and in the traditions of Jewish immigrants. Research articles on the medicinal properties of chicken soup have appeared in the scientific literature in the past ten years. Because no specific medicinal properties have been found in the chicken, scientists suspect the "active constituents" in chicken soup may be the garlic and/or onions that are commonly added.

make sure the water isn't too hot. This action lubricates the passages and helps expel phlegm.

Gargle hot water four times daily for ten minutes if a sore throat or earache accompanies your cold.

For general muscle and joint aches, take a fifteen minute hot hip bath (see "Cold Hip Bath," page 246). Follow with a brief cold shower and rapid, vigorous drying with a rough towel.

Here's how to treat a sore throat: Thoroughly soak a cotton cloth in cold water. Wring the cloth out and wrap it around your neck. Place a warm wool scarf over the cold cloth. Keep the cloths in place until the body has warmed up the cold cloth.

BUTTER: An old New England remedy for treating colds is to eat butter, either straight or melted in a cup of hot water or milk. Adding butter to hot tea is a remedy used as a cold preventive in the high altitudes of Nepal and Tibet. Cough syrups made with butter are also popular remedies in folk medicine.

Butter contains about 15 percent short- and medium-chain fatty acids, which, in laboratory tests, exhibit antibacterial, antifungal, and immune-stimulating properties. A single tablespoon of butter also contains more than 400 IU of vitamin A, about half the minimum daily requirement. Vitamin A also helps to maintain the health of the mucous membranes of the respiratory tract.

☞ DIRECTIONS: Eat 1 tablespoon of butter three or four times a day. Alternately, add 1 tablespoon of butter to 1 cup of hot tea. Let the butter melt so that it forms a thin layer across the top of the tea. Stir and drink.

❧ Constipation ❧

■ ■ ■

Constipation can mean either difficult or infrequent passage of the feces. Normal healthy bowels will produce between one and three bowel movements a day. Not an illness in itself, constipation, whether chronic or acute, can be the symptom of anything from a low-fiber diet to more serious illnesses. A medical checkup is warranted in any case of severe or persistent constipation. Constipation accompanied by nausea, vomiting, abdominal pain, or rectal bleeding or in the presence of any inflammatory bowel disease should never be treated with laxatives.

The most common cause of constipation in modern society is the modern diet. Constipation is classified by medical anthropologists H.C. Trowell and D.P. Burkitt as a "Western" condition, meaning that the condition does not appear in primitive people eating traditional diets—that is, until Western foods, such as sugar, white flour, and canned goods, are added.

Conventional physicians, alternative doctors, and folk healers alike all warn against the use of strong laxatives to force a bowel movement. From a medical point of view, if the constipation is due to a serious underlying disease, the laxative can cause injury and make that condition worse. Chronic use of strong laxatives also creates "laxative dependence"—a condition in which the bowels become so exhausted that they can no longer provide a normal bowel movement without the stimulation of more laxatives. Laxative dependence can also cause electrolyte (such as sodium and potassium) imbalances.

Conventional treatment for constipation, after a thorough investigation of the cause, is to increase fiber and liquids in the diet and to administer bulk laxatives such as psyllium husks. An increase in fruits and vegetables in the diet is also encouraged. Eat six or more servings of vegetables each day.

Many of the folk remedies for treating constipation include herbs that act as strong laxatives, but their use for more than seven to ten days is not warranted. Anything stronger than a bulk laxative (also called stool softeners) is contraindicated in pregnancy, however, because the same constituents that make the colon wall contract to

The Wisdom of Father Kneipp

During the late 1800s and early 1900s, German immigrants to New York and to other eastern states arrived with the book *My Water Cure* (English translation) written by Bavarian peasant priest and healer Father Sebastian Kneipp. Within thirty years of the book's arrival to this country, Kneipp's recommendations for diet, herbs, and water treatments were widespread. There was a monthly magazine promoting his opinions, and tens of thousands of medical professionals and lay people practiced his advice. Said Father Kneipp about laxative herbs and chemicals: "It will be noticed that I have not given the well-known and generally used laxatives, such as rhubarb, senna, epsom-salt, etc. And the reason? These in themselves harmless remedies are nevertheless too strong for me; help can be obtained by milder means. No one would chase a gnat or a flea with a gun." Simply increasing the amount of water we drink each day may help many disorders of the gastrointestinal tract.

produce a bowel movement can make the uterus contract as well. Stimulating laxatives are also contraindicated for use in children under 12 years of age.

Remedies

SENNA: Well known as a laxative, senna leaves *(Cassia senna),* most of which are imported from India, were brought to this country by European colonists. A North American variety of senna was used in the same way by Indians in eastern parts of the United States. Senna leaves have been used as a laxative by the Amish. Senna has been used for the same purpose in the folk medicine of New England, Appalachia, and the Southwest. Senna is also a component of some over-the-counter laxatives in North America and Europe. Senna is contraindicated in children, during pregnancy, and for

Appalachian Wisdom

Like Father Sebastian Kneipp (see sidebar, "The Wisdom of Father Kneipp," opposite), traditional Appalachian herbalist Tommie Bass cautioned against the habitual use of strong laxatives. Rather than avoid them, however, Bass recommended that a laxative be taken in small doses—doses that would soften the stool but not produce strong bowel movements. He cautioned that the use of low-dose laxatives was only for short term use, however.

Bass, who died in 1997, formulated and sold an herbal laxative mixture through his herb shop that combined small amounts of the stronger laxatives (senna and cascara sagrada) with more than a dozen other herbs. It was an herbal formula that seemed to work; users also noted improved overall digestion and liver function.

more than ten days at a time.

☞ DIRECTIONS: Do not use excessive amounts of senna. Place ¼ to ½ teaspoon of the dried crushed leaves or powder in a cup and fill with boiling water. Let steep seven to ten minutes. (A full teaspoon in a cup of tea is strong enough to produce abdominal cramping.)

CASCARA SAGRADA: At least 14 western Indian tribes have used cascara sagrada, or "sacred bark" *(Rhamnus purshiana),* as a laxative. Colonists learned its laxative effects from American Indian tribes in the Pacific Northwest. Its use spread to the folk medicine of the Southwest, New England, and Appalachia. Cascara sagrada is a common component of many of today's over-the-counter laxatives in North America.

Cascara sagrada bark must be aged for more than a year before it is used, or else it can induce vomiting. Usually the bark you buy in herb shops has been properly aged, though in rare instances, you might inadvertently purchase young bark. If the cascara leaves you feeling at all sick to your stomach, return it for a refund and shop somewhere else. The use of cascara sagrada is contraindicated in children, during pregnancy, and for more than ten days at a time. Do not use cascara sagrada in herbal formulas intended to help you lose weight.

☞ DIRECTIONS: Place 1 rounded teaspoon of the bark powder in a cup and fill with boiling water. Let steep until room temperature. Drinking a cup before bedtime will usually produce a bowel movement in the morning.

Alternately, place 1 ounce of aged cascara sagrada bark in a 1-quart jar, fill with boiling water, and let stand. The dose is 1 teaspoon in the morning and evening.

EPSOM SALTS: Epsom salts are composed of magnesium sulfate. The salts were first prepared from the waters of mineral springs in Epsom, England, where they were discovered in 1695. Their use as a commercial laxative spread quickly in the medicine of Europe; the salts remain popular there today. Epsom salts are now produced industrially and not from the springs in Epsom. The salts act as a laxative by drawing water out of the body and into the intestine. Epsom salts are listed in the folk medicine of New England and are widely used throughout North America as an over-the-counter laxative. Habitual use can cause dehydration and laxative dependence, however, so don't use Epsom salts for more than seven days.

☞ DIRECTIONS: Place 2 or 3 teaspoons of Epsom salts in a glass of warm water and drink. Do this once a day.

FLAX SEED: Flax seed (*Linum usitatissimum*) is a New England folk remedy for treating constipation. The remedy is also used among the Amish and by some Gypsies. Flax is a bulk laxative, meaning that its fiber absorbs water, expands, and provides bulk for bowel movements. Flax seed also contains high amounts of essential fatty acids. Flax seed works in the same way as psyllium seed, the chief component of the commercial bulk laxative Metamucil.

☞ DIRECTIONS: Take 2 teaspoons of flax seeds. Grind them in a coffee grinder and add to an 8-ounce glass of water. Let stand for half an hour and drink, seeds and all.

BONESET: In colonial days, boneset (*Eupatorium perfoliatum*) was one of the most often used medicinal herbs in North America. Ethnobotanical sources say that it was found hanging in the houses or barns of every "well regulated" household in the colonies. Hot boneset tea was taken to treat fevers, colds, and flu. Cold boneset tea was taken as a digestive tonic, and, sometimes, as a mild laxative.

Prunes vs. the FDA

In both New England and Appalachia, prunes or prune juice are recommended for treating constipation. Nineteenth century German immigrants also stood by the remedy. In fact, anyone who has had the misfortune of drinking too much prune juice can attest to the remedy's effectiveness!

The U.S. Food and Drug Administration (FDA) recently ordered American food companies to halt claims that their prune juice products acted as laxatives, however, because that effect had never been proven in clinical trials. This incident illustrates a common dilemma with many effective folk remedies in the United States—they remain outside the fold of official medicine because they have never been formally tested in a university, laboratory, or hospital setting.

The use of boneset as a laxative was recorded among the Mohawk Indians and persists today in the folk medicine of Appalachia. Always use the dried leaves, however, because fresh boneset contains mildly toxic substances. And don't exceed the recommended amounts, because larger amounts can cause nausea or induce vomiting, one of its older medicinal uses.

☞ DIRECTIONS: Place 1 teaspoon of dried boneset leaves in a cup and fill with boiling water. Cover and let stand until cooled to room temperature. Drink ¼ cup three times a day for up to five days.

SESAME SEEDS: According to the Amish, sesame seeds have a laxative effect. Chinese folk medicine claims the same. The seeds are nutritious and also contain about 55 percent oil, which helps to moisten the intestines in those suffering from dry constipation.

☞ DIRECTIONS: Eat up to ½ ounce of sesame

Enemas

The use of enemas is occasionally mentioned as a treatment for constipation in the literature of folk medicine. It was a widespread practice among American Indians and persists today among the Seventh Day Adventists. Overuse of enemas can be injurious to the bowels, however, because the enemas wash away normal protective mucus, deplete the body of electrolyte salts, and possibly introduce foreign or irritating matter into the bowels.

seeds a day. Grind fresh seeds in a coffee grinder and sprinkle on food like a condiment.

HOT WATER: A remedy from New England also mentioned by the Amish is to drink a cup of hot water in the morning. Similar practices, slightly modified, appear throughout the world. In the folk medicine of India, the prescription is to drink a quart of room temperature water in the morning. German followers of the water cures of Father Sebastian Kneipp (see sidebar, "The Wisdom of Father Kneipp," page 122) take the water hot in 1-tablespoon doses every half hour all day.

Drinking water in the morning to produce a bowel movement has a solid physiological basis. An internal digestive reflex causes the bowels to contract and move the stool in the direction of the anus in response to stretching of the stomach. The stretch reflex can be triggered most easily in the morning, when the stomach is most contracted. Drinking water can trigger this stretch reflex.

☞ DIRECTIONS: Drink 1 to 3 cups of hot water first thing in the morning on an empty stomach.

❦ Coughs ❦

▦ ▦ ▦

Coughing can result from inhaling dust, dirt, or irritating fumes; from breathing icy air; or from mistakenly drawing food into the airways. It can also be caused by mucus and other secretions from such respiratory disorders as the common cold, influenza, pneumonia, or tuberculosis.

The respiratory passages in the throat and lungs are constantly kept moist by a layer of mucus. This mucus traps small particles, viruses, bacteria, dust, pollen, or other materials. The surfaces of these passageways are so sensitive to touch that any irritation there will cause a cough reflex—a reflex that expels the irritating matter at velocities as high as 100 miles an hour. This reflex usually removes any loose mucus or other matter. A cough is thus a healthy healing mechanism, necessary to remove allergens, viruses, bacteria, or foreign matter from the respiratory tract.

Both pharmaceutical drugs and folk remedies aid coughs in several ways. Some folk remedies, like the herbs licorice or marshmallow, are demulcents; they moisten and soothe the throat and bronchial tract, reducing the cough reflex by reducing irritation of the tissues. Others, such as garlic or honey, are expectorants and work by promoting the secretion of fresh mucus, which aids the body in washing out irritants. Finally, cherry bark and the over-the-counter drug dextromethorphan, are respiratory sedatives. They act on the nervous system to reduce the cough reflex. Such a reduction is appropriate for short-term use when an unproductive cough interferes with sleep or is overly exhausting. Sedatives are not appropriate for productive coughs with a lot of mucus, however, because the cough is necessary to clear the lungs of mucus.

According to the Public Citizen Health Research Group, dextromethorphan is the best cough suppressant to use. It is a component of many over-the-counter cough remedies and syrups. The Public Citizen Health Research Group recommends purchasing generic dextromethorphan at a pharmacy or taking a product containing only dextromethorphan, which will suppress a cough for about twelve hours and allow a good night's sleep.

The actions of cough remedies, even the over-the-counter pharmaceutical types, are difficult to prove. There is no scientific evidence supporting that these herbs effectively treat coughs, probably due to the difficulty in accurately measuring expectoration.

Remedies

WILD CHERRY BARK: The use of wild cherry bark *(Prunus serotina)* to

Pass the Honey

Honey has been used in traditional Chinese medicine for more than 2,000 years. It is used for conditions ranging from asthma, cough, and chronic bronchitis to stomachache, constipation, chronic sinus congestion, canker sores, and burns. A folk remedy from China for treating coughs calls for a tablespoon of honey in hot water. Expectorant syrups made from honey are widespread throughout the folk traditions of the world, and appear in the folk medicine of every region in the United States. Honey is a natural expectorant, promoting the flow of mucus.

treat coughs was taught to the British colonists by the Cherokee and the Iroquois eastern Indian tribes. Other tribes throughout North America have used various wild cherry species in the same way. Use of the bark became very popular throughout the United States in the 19th century. Wild cherry bark is still used as a cough remedy in the folk medicine of the Amish, New Englanders, and residents of the Southwest. It is also used in contemporary North American and European medical herbalism. "Wild cherry" cough drops are available in stores today, although they are now made with artificial flavors instead of actual wild cherry bark.

The bark's constituent prunasin reduces the cough reflex, so wild cherry is classified as a cough suppressant. Thus, it requires the same cautions as the over-the-counter medication dextromethorphan. Prunasin is a potentially toxic compound. But, if taken as a tea in the correct quantities, adults are safe using it. All cases of toxicity from wild cherry have occurred in children eating the fruit—called "choke cherries"—along with the toxic pits, which contain large amounts of prunasin and related compounds.

Wild cherry has expectorant and demulcent properties, too, so this herb is like a complete cough formula all rolled up in one. Wild cherry bark is especially suited to dry, irritating coughs. Combining it with another demulcent will further improve its effects.

☞ DIRECTIONS: Place 1 tablespoon of wild cherry bark and an equal part of licorice root in 1 pint of water. Boil for five minutes, remove from heat, sweeten with ½ cup of honey. Let stand until the mixture cools to room temperature. The dose is ¼ cup, no more than five times a day. To remain on the side of caution, don't give cherry bark to children under the age of twelve. Adults shouldn't take cherry bark for more than three consecutive days. Women should avoid cherry bark altogether if they are pregnant or nursing.

FLAX SEEDS: New Englanders and residents of other eastern states use boiled flax seeds (*Linum usitatissimum*) to treat coughs. Boiled flax seeds make a thick demulcent that is soothing to the throat and bronchial tract.

☞ DIRECTIONS: Boil 2 or 3 tablespoons of flax seeds in 1 cup of water for a few minutes, until the water becomes gooey. Strain. Add equal parts of honey and lemon juice. For a dry irritable cough that's not producing much mucus, take 1-tablespoon doses as needed.

BLACK PEPPER: A remedy for coughs from New England, which also appears in Chinese folk medicine, is black pepper (*Piper nigrum*). The irritating properties of black pepper stimulate circulation and the flow of mucus. Black pepper works best on coughs producing a thick mucus; it is inappropriate for a dry, irritable cough with little expectoration.

☞ DIRECTIONS: Place 1 teaspoon of black pepper and 1 tablespoon of honey in a cup and fill with boiling water. Let steep for ten to fifteen minutes. Take small sips as needed.

MUSTARD SEED: An old New England cough remedy calls for mustard seed. Mustard is also used for treating coughs in the folk medicine of China. Mustard has irritating sulfur-containing compounds that stimulate the flow of mucus. Like pepper, above, it is only appropriate for congested productive coughs with plenty of mucus present. It will irritate a dry cough and make it worse.

☞ DIRECTIONS: Crush 1 teaspoon of mustard seeds or grind them in a coffee grinder. Place the seeds in a cup and fill with warm water. Steep for fifteen minutes. (The

Coughs, Dry and Wet

A cough is a healthy healing mechanism, necessary to remove allergens, viruses, or bacteria from the respiratory tract. Mucus traps these invading and irritating substances. The secretion of the mucus and its expulsion from your body when you cough is part of the body's healing process.

With some coughs—such as "wet" coughs—plenty of mucus is present, but the mucus is thick, gummy, and hard to expel. Acrid, irritating, and stimulating herbs are helpful for treating these types of coughs because they stimulate the flow of new, clean mucus, which helps expel the old.

"Dry" coughs typically accompany the flu. Acrid and stimulating herbs only irritate dry coughs further because there is little mucus to expel. To treat a dry cough, try a soothing herb such as slippery elm, mallow, or licorice.

expectorant compounds are not released until the mustard seeds are crushed or broken and allowed to sit in water or some other medium for about fifteen minutes.) Take in ¼-cup doses throughout the day.

GARLIC: Early medical records from all over the globe show that garlic (*Allium sativum*) was used as a treatment for coughs and bronchial conditions. Garlic and honey syrups are standard cough treat-ments in the folk medicine of the Southwest today.

Garlic was acknowledged as an expectorant in the National Formulary of the United States from 1916 until 1936. Garlic is not appropriate for treating dry, unproductive coughs, however. It is best for treating coughs that are producing mucus.

☞ DIRECTIONS: Put 1 pound of sliced garlic in 1 quart of boiling water; let it soak for ten to twelve minutes, keeping the water warm (but not boiling). Strain and add 4 pounds of honey. Strain and bottle the syrup. When you feel congested, take 1 teaspoonful.

ONION SYRUP: In *American Folk Medicine,* folklorist Clarence Meyer suggests taking a honey-and-onion syrup for treating coughs. Onions have anti-inflammatory properties that may reduce throat irritation, and honey is a natural expectorant, promoting the free flow of mucus. Onions also contain the antiviral constituent protocatechuic acid, which attacks viruses, including the one that may be causing the cough.

☞ DIRECTIONS: Chop 5 or 6 white onions and place them in a double boiler. Add ½ cup of honey and the juice of 1 lemon and cook at lowest heat possible for several hours. Strain the mixture and take by the tablespoon as needed—from every half an hour to every few hours.

HOREHOUND: A folk remedy for coughs from contemporary New Mexico is horehound *(Marrubium vulgare),* a European plant that arrived in North America with both the Spanish and northern European colonists. Horehound has been used to treat coughs in European folk medicine since the time of the ancient Greeks. It was an official cough remedy in the *United States Pharmacopoeia* between 1840 and 1910, and it remains an approved medicine for coughs by the German government today.

Horehound stimulates the flow of mucus, and is indicated for use in unproductive coughs. Horehound can be irritating and increase the discomfort of dry coughs, however.

☞ DIRECTIONS: Place 1 tablespoon of dried horehound in a cup and fill with boiling water. Cover and let steep for fifteen minutes. Sweeten with honey. Drink in ½-cup doses as often as desired.

continued on page 138

Animal Cures Down on the Farm

▩ ▩ ▩

Folk medicine has always made use of materials that are readily on hand, including common foods, such as honey and vinegar, and plants. Animals, numerous and easily accessible in rural life, have also figured prominently into the folk remedies of all cultures. But, while patients use them in the hopes of bringing about health benefits, the animals usually get the short end of the stick.

Some reported animal remedies appear so unreal that it's hard to believe they were ever really used. For example, one man in Illinois claimed that a woman could avoid headaches by binding a live toad to her forehead. Toads are commonly used in remedies, but, as a long-term preventive, this seems more like a cruel joke, not a practical recommendation!

At the other end of the spectrum there are remedies that are very similar to the conventional treatments we use today. For instance, mutton tallow—the fat from sheep—was used in folk remedies to prevent and treat chapped hands and lips. In fact, all sorts of animal fats have long been used as emollients to soften and soothe skin. Today we use lanolin, an oil obtained from sheep wool, for the same purpose.

DOGS AND CATS: Cats and dogs evoke great loyalty from their human owners. Perhaps that is the reason these animals are not used in folk remedies as often as other domesticated animals. Nonetheless, there have been some uses reported. In the Southwest, it is said that if a Mexican Chihuahua sleeps on your bed, you will be cured of rheumatism. (The same has been said about

Hog Magic

Hogs are famous for being completely consumable—right down to their squeal! So it is not surprising that even hogs' feet can be used in a tea (with pine buds and resin) for respiratory ailments. But some cures involving hogs were surprisingly magical. For example, a sore neck could be treated by rubbing it against a tree where a hog had rubbed; mumps were treated by rubbing the swollen areas with marrow from a hog jaw or by rubbing an ailing child's jaw on a pig trough. And, if the patient was too ill to get to the trough, the hog was brought to the sickroom so the child could rub his jaw directly on the hog's jowl!

guinea pigs, especially by the Slavic and German Americans.) For some, the belief is that the remedy works by transferring the rheumatism from the patient to the animal. Others believe that the remedy is advantageous to the health of the animal and the owner alike. Chihuahuas kept in the house are also said to prevent asthma. This belief probably originates from the fact that the dander from furry pets is an allergen, and Chihuahuas have very little fur.

The few reported remedies involving cats are less favorable to the animals' well-being. In Georgia, it has been said that to cure shingles (a painful infection by the herpes zoster virus that is accompanied by skin eruptions) a person should rub the blood of a black cat on the inflamed area. An even more gruesome treatment for shingles, found both in the Midwest and among Pennsylvania Germans, says to paint the shingles with the blood from the stump of a black cat's tail! An African-American remedy uses the black cat's blood on a lump of sugar to be taken internally.

In the United States and Europe, it is widely believed that cat's fur worn against the skin will absorb arthritic pain, and, as recently as the 1960s, cats' pelts were sold in French drugstores for this purpose. In Utah, wearing cat's fur against the skin is believed by some to cure tuberculosis and pneumonia.

CHICKENS: Farm animals figure more prominently into folk medicine, probably because butchering is inevitable for many of these animals. Chickens are used quite prominently in folk medicine—and we should remember that chicken soup is still widely reputed to have healing properties. Most medicinal uses of chickens have been much less savory and far from kosher, however! One treatment for colitis (inflammation of the large intestine) is a "tea" made by steeping a whole chicken— complete with feathers—in water. Some believe chicken blood, especially the blood of a black chicken, has healing qualities. A cure for shingles from Georgia involves pulling the head off a live black hen and holding the carcass so that the blood flows over the affected body part. A cloth is wrapped around the patient to catch the blood and the blood is then used as a dressing. The cloth is left in place until it falls off on its own accord—at which time the shingles will be gone. The same use of a black chicken's blood, for both shingles and hives, has been reported in remedies from the Midwest.

In some remedies it is the blood and meat that affect the cure, as in the following treatment for snake bite, reported in Illinois. A chicken was split and one half of the raw carcass was tied over the bite area to draw out the poison. (While this practice may sound bizarre, realize that many people still believe that blood can be drawn from a bruise by holding a raw steak against it, especially in the case of a black eye.) A treatment from

Maryland used additional magical elements: The raw split chicken (preferably black in color) was put on the feet of a feverish patient, while the chicken's feathers were burnt under the patient's bed. Finally, also from Maryland, a remedy that even the chicken could survive: Children with chicken pox were put in front of a chicken house so that chickens could fly over them. Like many animal remedies, this one probably has its origins in the belief that the disease can be transferred from the patient to the animal.

HORSES AND MULES: At one time there were almost as many horses and mules as there were chickens, and the animals were equally valued in folk medicine. However, while chickens were expendable, horses and mules were not—most of the remedies left these larger animals completely intact! For example, in Georgia it has been said that sore eyes can be cured by washing them in a mule's watering trough, and, in both California and Utah, it has been reported that a toothache can be cured by kissing a mule. But most often it is the breath of horses and mules that seems to be the most powerful. In Illinois, it is said that kissing the nostrils of a mule will cure catarrh and that tonsillitis is cured by having a horse blow in the patient's mouth. In California, if the horse is a full-bred stallion, his breath can be used to cure whooping cough. Other horse and mule remedies seem purely magical, such as the idea that sleeping in the hay with horses will relieve tuberculosis or that children's respiratory illnesses can be cured by simply being passed under the belly of a mule or horse.

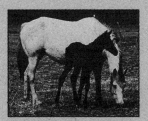

Remedies using horses usually left the animals completely intact.

OSHA SYRUP: Osha *(Ligusticum porteri)* was a medicinal plant popular among American Indians and settlers residing in the higher elevations of the Rocky Mountains. Osha has a hot acrid taste, and its constituents possesses both expectorant and antiviral properties. American Indians of the area believed that osha has the power to repel evil spirits.

☞ DIRECTIONS: Grind 1 ounce of osha root in a coffee grinder. Heat 1 pint of honey in a pot, and add the osha root. Simmer slowly until the honey becomes thick. Leave the root in the honey and let cool to room temperature. Do not strain. Take 1-tablespoon doses of the syrup four to six times a day as desired.

MULLEIN: Did you know you can make a cough syrup with the leaves of the mullein plant? Mullein *(Verbascum thapsus)* came to North America with the European colonists and is now naturalized throughout the United States and Canada. Its use as a cough medicine was quickly adopted by several American Indian tribes, including the Mohegan, Delaware, Cherokee, Creek, and Navaho. It appears today in the folk medicine of Appalachia and the Southwest. Mullein was an official cough medicine in the *United States Pharmacopoeia* from 1888 until 1936 and remains an approved medicine for cough in Germany. Recent research shows that mullein tea also may have an antiviral effect against the influenza virus.

☞ DIRECTIONS: Place ½ pound of mullein leaves in a 1-quart jar. Fill with boiling water and let cool to room temperature. Strain and add honey until the mixture has the consistency of a syrup. The dose is 1 tablespoon as needed.

SLIPPERY ELM: Slippery elm bark *(Ulmus fulva)* has a slimy mucilaginous texture that is soothing to inflamed tissues in the mouth and throat. It is

That's Pine

Pine bark or pine pitch (congealed pine sap) was a commonly used American Indian cough treatment. The practice also dates back to the ancient Greeks. Colonists in the eastern states, whether they brought the practice with them from Europe or learned it from the American Indians, used pine pitch and pine bark as well—often adding it to their cough formulas or syrups. One simple syrup from folklorist Clarence Meyer's *American Folk Medicine* calls for a tea of the inner bark of pine, sweetened with honey and made into a syrup. Pine oils are extremely stimulating, however, and the bark or sap should never be used on dry, irritable coughs.

ideally suited to treat a cough that accompanies a sore throat. Slippery elm cough lozenges have been sold in the United States since the late 1800s. It was an official cough remedy in the *United States Pharmacopoeia* from 1820 until 1930. It is used to treat coughs in Appalachia today.

☞ DIRECTIONS: Stir 1 ounce of slippery elm bark powder and 3 tablespoons of honey into 1 pint of boiling water. Let stand for half an hour. Strain and take 1-tablespoon doses as desired.

MALLOW: For a dry or inflamed cough high in the respiratory tract that's accompanied by a sore throat, a tea made from marshmallow (*Althea officinalis*) or hollyhock (*Althea rosea*) and honey may bring relief. Both plants have been used in traditional European herbalism at least since the time of the ancient Greeks. The plants came to North America as garden plants and are still used today to treat coughs in professional medical herbalism.

Dried marshmallow root contains up to one-third

mucilage. Marshmallow is also expectorant, so the double action of the plant mucilage and its ability to increase natural mucus will help soothe the inflamed membranes of the throat.

Hollyhock flowers may be used instead of marshmallow root. The 19th century German herbal *My Water Cure* (English translation), a popular book among German immigrants in the United States, says, "Among the flowers in the garden, hollyhock must not be missing. When the good creator painted its blossoms, so pleasing to the eye, he poured a drop of medicinal sap into the paint for every petal."

☞ DIRECTIONS: Cover 1 ounce of chopped marshmallow root with 1 pint of boiling water and let steep until cool. Add 2 tablespoons of honey to a cup of the tea and sip as often as desired throughout the day. Also, try placing a handful of hollyhock flowers and a handful of dried mullein leaves in a 1-pint canning jar. Fill with boiling water, cover, and let stand overnight. Strain, and sweeten with honey. Take ¼-cup doses as desired.

LICORICE: Licorice root *(Glycyrrhiza glabra)* has been used to treat coughs and bronchial problems in many traditions throughout the world. It is listed in several 19th century folk remedy collections from the eastern United States. It was an official medicine in the *United States Pharmacopoeia* from 1820 until 1975; it was recommended as a flavoring agent and a demulcent and expectorant for cough syrups. (Most licorice candy in the United States is really flavored with anise oil.)

☞ DIRECTIONS: Cut 1 ounce of licorice sticks into slices, and add to 1 quart of boiling water. Steep for twenty-four hours. Drink throughout the day, adding honey to taste.

GINGER: Several North American Indian tribes,

including the Allegheny and Montagnais, used wild North American ginger *(Asarum canadensis)* for treating coughs. Ginger is commonly used today in Chinese folk medicine. Ginger contains both anti-inflammatory and anti-spasmodic chemical constituents.

☞ DIRECTIONS: Thinly slice a fresh ginger root (about the size of your thumb). Place in 1 quart of water. Bring to a boil. Simmer in a covered pot on the lowest possible heat for thirty minutes. Let cool for thirty minutes more. Strain and drink ½ to 1 cup, sweetened with honey, as often as desired. Ginger can be irritating to hot, dry, unproductive coughs and should thus be avoided when such a cough is present.

ELECAMPANE: Elecampane *(Inula helenium),* has been used to treat coughs and bronchitis since the time of the ancient Greeks. (Its Latin name, *helenium,* comes from Helen of Troy, who supposedly was holding the plant as she left her home for Troy.) A native plant of south-eastern Europe, elecampane came to North America with the European colonists. Its use for coughs was quickly adopted by the American Indians, and it is still included today as a cough medicine in the folklore of the Iroquois. It is also used in contemporary Chinese medicine for the same purposes. Elecampane is a mild expectorant, so it may be irritating to a dry cough.

☞ DIRECTIONS: Place 1 tablespoon of dried elecampane root in 2 cups of water and simmer for twenty minutes in a well-covered pot. Drink 2 to 3 cups a day.

BUTTERY SYRUPS: Adding butter to a hot cough syrup is common throughout North American folklore, especially in the eastern and northeastern states. Butter may be soothing to the tissues because of its texture, and some of its constituents may also be beneficial. Butter contains vitamin A, which helps to regenerate mucous membranes. It also contains short- and medium-chain fatty acids, which possess antimicrobial properties. It may thus help kill germs in the mouth and throat that may be responsible for causing the cough in the first place. The recipe below is from *American Folk Medicine*. (It has been adapted to substitute honey for sugar.)

☞ DIRECTIONS: Mix equal parts of butter, vinegar, honey, and hot water. Add a pinch of cinnamon. Simmer for thirty to forty minutes to make a thick syrup.

HYDROTHERAPY: Hydrotherapy has its roots in the German tradition of naturopathy; it was brought to North America by immigrants near the turn of the 20th century. Here's a hydrotherapy treatment

Great Expectoration

For a dry cough or one accompanied by thick (rather than watery) mucous secretions, be sure to drink enough liquids. Water is a natural expectorant, so drink plenty of it—whether in the form of water, soups, or teas. A Seventh Day Adventist treatment calls for taking a sip of water every time you cough.

You can also moisten the respiratory tract with steam from a vaporizer or a hot shower or simply by inhaling steam from hot water running in the sink.

from New England for treating coughs.

☞ DIRECTIONS: Soak a cotton cloth or cotton scarf in cold water. Wring it out and wrap it around the front of the neck below the ears, carefully avoiding contact with the back of the neck. Wrap a warm wool scarf around the wet cloth and lie down. The cold cloth will attract circulation to the area, soothing the cough and promoting healing.

❧ Depression ❧

▣ ▣ ▣

Depression is a psychological condition characterized by prolonged sadness, combined with other symptoms, including persistent low, anxious, or "empty" feelings, decreased energy, loss of interest or pleasure in usual activities, sleep disturbances, and feelings of hopelessness. Depression may be due to an imbalance or lack of certain necessary brain chemicals.

Some types of depression run in families, indicating that a biological vulnerability to the condition can be inherited. Psychological makeup also plays a role in vulnerability to depression. People who have low self-esteem, who consistently view themselves and the world with pessimism, or who are readily overwhelmed by stress are prone to depression. A serious loss, chronic illness, difficult relationship, financial problem, or unwelcome change in life patterns can also trigger a depressive episode.

Depression can occur because of normal chemical changes in the body. Two examples are premenstrual depression and postpartum depression, both thought to be linked to female hormonal activities. In addition, certain drugs, including oral contraceptives, alcohol, and some sedatives, may cause a side effect of depression in some people. Certain infections (including influenza) can depress a person's mood, as can over- or underproduction of hormones by the outer layer of the adrenal gland, or a deficiency of vitamin B_{12}. Scientific evidence has also linked some forms of depression to deficiencies of the vitamins biotin, folic acid, pantothenic acid, pyridoxine, riboflavin, thiamine, vitamin C, and vitamin E. Deficiencies in the minerals calcium, copper, iron, magnesium, potassium, and zinc can also cause depression. (In fact, deficiencies of magnesium and zinc alone can cause symptoms that can lead to a diagnosis of depression. According to the U.S. Department of Agriculture, the average American does not consume the minimum daily requirement of either mineral.) So, before taking antidepressant drugs, patients with mild depression would be wise to undergo a thorough screening of their nutritional status.

Traditional societies are less likely than we are to report depression in their literature because they are more likely to consume a whole-food, nutrient-dense diet and to get sufficient exercise. Weston Price, a nutritional anthropologist who studied traditional societies around the world in the 1930s, found that primitive people consuming a traditional diet take in from three to ten times the vitamin and mineral content found in modern diets.

Very few folk remedies appear for depression in folk literature; the word itself is a 20th century medical term. Older texts are more likely to refer to depression as melancholy (depressive mood), neurasthenia (nervous exhaustion), malaise (profound fatigue), possession, or witchcraft.

Depression can be very serious. Depression with thoughts of suicide requires immediate medical attention. Conventional treatment for depression includes taking an antidepressant and, sometimes, participating in psychotherapy.

Remedies

ST. JOHN'S WORT: St. John's wort is a common meadowland plant that has been used as a medicine for centuries. (It is mentioned in early European and Slavic herbals.) The genus name *Hypericum* is from the Latin *hyper,* meaning "above," and *icon,* meaning "spirit." The herb was hung over doorways to ward off evil spirits or burned to protect and sanctify an area. German immigrants to the United States at the turn of the century used it as a digestive herb for "melancholy."

St. John's wort is reported to relieve anxiety and tension and to act as an antidepressant. The herb is an approved medicine in Germany. With long-term use, hypericin, one of the constituents, may make the skin of a few individuals more sensitive to sunlight, however.

☞ DIRECTIONS: Purchase St. John's wort from a health food store, herb shop, or pharmacy. Take as directed. Alternately, you can purchase a St. John's wort tincture at a health food store or herb shop. A good quality tincture will be dark red in color.

For a more traditional formula, try this Gypsy "soul-refreshing tonic": Gather properly identified wild St. John's wort leaves and flowers, enough to fill a loosely packed pint or quart jar. To follow ancient traditions, harvest them on St. John's day, the day after the summer solstice. (You can do this in most parts of the country, but at higher elevations the flowers will not yet be in bloom, so you'll have to wait a little longer to try this remedy.) Cover the leaves and flowers with 90 proof liquor. Let stand for one cycle of the moon, shaking the bottle daily. Strain and rebottle. Take 10 to 20 drops daily.

CALIFORNIA POPPY: California poppy (*Eschscholtzia californica*) was used as a treatment of the nervous system by the Costanoan Indians. California poppy eventually made its way into European medicine, and today pharmaceutical preparations of the herb are prescribed by physicians in Germany for nervous disorders, including mild depression. The Germans consider the herb to be so gentle that it is sometimes prescribed for treating mild emotional disorders in children. (Although it bears the name "poppy," the herb is not a narcotic and contains no morphine or codeine-type alkaloids.)

California poppy is not readily available in the herb trade, but it grows freely in the western United States and is a common garden plant in other areas. Do not use during pregnancy or while nursing.

☞ DIRECTIONS: Pick some California poppies, using the stems, leaves, and flowers of the plant. Let them dry in a warm place, out of direct sunlight. Place 1 teaspoon of the dried herb in a cup and fill the cup with boiling water. Cover and let steep for twenty minutes. Strain

The Sluggish Liver

Sluggish liver function has little meaning in North American conventional medicine. But "bile deficiency," the physiological equivalent of sluggish liver function, is commonly treated in both French and German contemporary medicine. Contemporary French physicians attribute conditions such as fatigue, physical sluggishness, and headache to this low-grade liver dysfunction.

In traditional Western medicine, melancholy, an older term for depression, was associated with sluggish liver function. The connection between liver function and depression is also seen in contemporary Chinese medicine. In fact, Chinese herbs, foods, and formulas designed to stimulate the liver are frequently prescribed for treating depression. Several of the remedies in this section are traditional treatments for sluggish liver, including St. John's wort, wormwood, boneset, dandelion, and increased exercise.

How Depressing

Many people with borderline depression turn to alcohol or recreational drugs to lift their mood. But alcohol is a "pick-me-up" that might just "bring you down."

Alcohol, the most popular drug of choice in modern society, is a depressant. Alcohol dulls the brain and the nervous system, slowing reactions and making drinkers feel relaxed and tranquilized. It can also lower inhibitions and make a person aggressive or hostile. In higher doses, it may block memory and impair concentration, judgment, coordination, and emotional reactions.

The liver is one of the primary targets of chronic alcohol abuse. In alcoholic hepatitis, liver cells are damaged or destroyed as a result of recent heavy drinking. Prolonged excessive drinking can lead to alcoholic cirrhosis, a condition in which large areas of the liver are destroyed or scarred. Liver damage is extremely serious and may be life-threatening.

Chronic depression and anxiety are common in habitual drinkers. In fact, one or two glasses of alcohol a day may cause or contribute to depression in some individuals.

and drink 1 to 3 cups a day, as desired.

DANDELION AND MOLASSES: A traditional treatment for "bilious" depression, according to folklorist Clarence Meyer in his book *American Folk Medicine,* combines dandelion root with molasses.

This "double-duty" treatment may help depression associated with a sluggish liver while, at the same time, restore mineral deficiencies that contribute to fatigue and low energy. Blackstrap molasses contains high amounts of essential minerals—a *continued on page 151*

Illnesses Unique to Folk Medicine

※ ※ ※

The most obvious difference between folk medicine and modern medicine is the existence of entirely different kinds of sicknesses. Often called "folk illnesses," some of the best-known examples of such illnesses in the United States are found among Latino ethnic groups. But all cultures have traditions about certain sicknesses. Some of these traditions vary from modern medicine only in the way that the illnesses are diagnosed and explained. For example, in some traditions, folk healers will diagnose cancer as being caused by a curse.

Other folk illnesses are more difficult to equate with a recognized medical condition. This is especially true in the case of psychiatric illnesses. For example, among the Hopi Indians, there exists an illness that is called "heart broken," but can also be translated as "heart is dying." The symptoms of the illness seem mostly physical and are caused by the loss of an important relationship. Psychiatrists have identified this condition as one of five different kinds of emotional problems that can be equated with what mainstream medicine terms as depression.

Other folk illnesses seem to have no equivalent at all in Western society. These illnesses are called "culture-bound syndromes," and some anthropologists and psychiatrists believe that they are actually produced by the culture in which they are found.

CULTURE-BOUND SYNDROMES
One of the best examples of a culture-bound syndrome is latah. Latah is an Indonesian word that refers to a person

who behaves in some very specific and bizarre ways when startled. The person who is latah will briefly obey commands (even ridiculous ones), repeat anything shouted at them, and often say dirty or blasphemous words. At one time scholars believed that this condition was caused by Indonesian child-rearing practices. But, as it turns out, the same condition is found in many cultures, just under different names. For instance, among French-Canadians living in New England, people who respond this way when startled are called "jumpers." Latah is caused by being especially sensitive to being startled—and such people are found in every society. People in some cultures have traditional knowledge of this condition while others, like most of American society, do not. This suggests that culture does not so much cause these conditions as it shapes the way that they are experienced and understood.

SPIRITUAL MEANS

Folk illnesses usually have a prominent spiritual element, and they are typically treated by spiritual means. This spiritual element is one factor that differentiates certain folk illnesses from Western medical diagnoses, since Western medicine has excluded spiritual explanations and diagnoses for centuries.

Soul-loss illnesses, such as Mexican susto, make up a kind of folk illness where folk tradition's knowledge may be beyond the learning of scientific medicine. Susto may actually be based on local knowledge of near-death experiences and the emotional changes that can follow, something that psychiatrists are only beginning to investigate and understand (see "Curanderismo," page 312).

In addition to experiencing the loss of your soul, you could also suffer from any of the folk illnesses thought to be caused by spirits. An example of a spirit-caused illness is ghost sickness, which is found among a number of American Indian tribes. This illness involves a preoccu-

pation with the dead, feelings of suffocation, and, sometimes, even a loss of consciousness.

THE PHYSICAL ELEMENT

Some folk illnesses seem very physical, but they differ
from sicknesses described by modern medicine. An
example is áwachse, or "liver grown" (the common English translation). This ailment is best known in the United
States among the Pennsylvania Germans. It is also known
in Germany, England, and the American South. Áwachse
means "to grow together." It is believed that the disorder
is caused by the liver becoming attached to the ribs or
other parts of the body cavity. The condition is believed to
be most common in young children, especially after they
have been exposed to strong wind, kept outside too long,
or been "shaken up" in travel.

In the American South, the most common symptom of
liver grown is a child's failure to thrive. The treatments
for this condition include magical remedies as well as the
act of stretching the arms and legs behind the child's back
to loosen the liver. Among the Pennsylvania Germans, a
definite diagnosis comes from feeling the lower chest. If
the child has áwachse the healer will feel the flesh pulled
inward. For the Pennsylvania Germans, most treatments
for this disorder involve passing the child under or
through something: beneath a bramble bush or through a
warm horse collar.

Some researchers have suggested that culture-bound
disorders may be found in modern Western culture. Thus,
it is important for doctors and nurses to be aware of the
existence of folk illnesses. When there is understanding
between patient and physician, it is possible to incorpo-
rate culturally sanctioned healing into medical treatment,
yielding more humane care. In addition, these folk illnesses are useful to us: They represent bodies of knowledge that Western medicine has yet to recognize.

tablespoon contains more than 15 percent of the daily requirement of calcium, magnesium, iron, potassium, copper, and manganese.

☞ DIRECTIONS: Simmer 4 ounces of dandelion root in 2 quarts of water until half of the water is gone. Strain and add a cup of molasses. Take 1 tablespoon three to four times a day, twenty minutes before meals. Try the treatment for three weeks, then take a break for a week or two.

WORMWOOD: Wormwood *(Artemisia absinthum)* has been widely used to treat "melancholy" in European medicine. Also, at least seven North American Indian tribes used it as "witchcraft medicine"—the symptoms of possession and depression may have been similarly interpreted.

In addition to its mild antidepressant effects, wormwood increases the secretion of bile in the liver and has anti-inflammatory properties.

Wormwood may be toxic, however, if taken for long periods of time.

☞ DIRECTIONS: Purchase a wormwood tincture at a health food store or herb shop. Using a dropper, take 15 drops of the tincture two or three times a day for two to three weeks.

OATS: Oats *(Avena sativa)* are a folk remedy for neurasthenia, or "nervous exhaustion," which is an old term for depression. At the turn of the century, the use of oats to treat nervous exhaustion was widespread among the Eclectic physicians, a school of physicians who used herbal remedies.

Oats are highly nutritious. In fact, one cup of

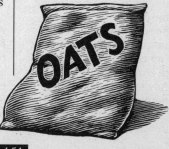

oats contains 26 grams of protein, 4 grams of essential fatty acids, 7.4 milligrams of iron, 276 milligrams of magnesium, 0.5 milligrams of copper, 6 milligrams of zinc, 7.1 milligrams of manganese, and 97 micrograms of folic acid—values that are more than half the recommended dietary allowance for each of these nutrients. Clinical research has demonstrated that oats may also aid in withdrawal from addictions.

☞ DIRECTIONS: Place 1 cup of oats in 3 cups of water and simmer for forty minutes in a covered pot. Add molasses or honey to taste. Pour off the liquid and save—you can drink it during the day. Eat the remaining gruel.

WATER TREATMENT: A hydrotherapy treatment for depression that was popular among German immigrants at the turn of the century, and remains in use by the Seventh Day Adventists today, is the neutral bath. In a neutral bath, the patient relaxes in water that is kept within a degree or two above body temperature for twenty to forty minutes. Water immersion has been shown in clinical trials to lower the circulating levels of stress hormones in the body. The treatment itself may be as old as the ancient Romans, who used hot, cold, or neutral water to treat medical conditions.

☞ DIRECTIONS: Run a tub of bathwater at 96–98°F. Soak in the bath for twenty to forty minutes. Repeat most days as part of your daily routine for three to six weeks.

WORK ON YOURSELF: If you are depressed, the Amish suggest you should "work on yourself." The same advice is recorded in the folk literature of the southern Appalachians.

A modern version of this view is psychotherapy. Fortunately, in the last two decades, some of the stigma of "seeing a therapist" has fallen away, and most people today view participating in therapy as a sign of healthy growth

Adaptogens:
Asian Remedies for Depression

Adaptogens are plants that help the body respond to sources of stress, including such things as overwork, lack of sleep, and overexposure to the elements. Three of the key symptoms of depression are fatigue, appetite loss, and lowering of sexual libido, and adaptogens are used in the traditional medicine of Asia (and in Chinatowns throughout North America) to treat all three of these symptoms. The two most famous of the Asian adaptogens are Asian ginseng (*Panax ginseng*) and Siberian ginseng (*Eleutherococcus senticosus*). A wide array of products containing the plants are available in health foods stores, herb shops, pharmacies, supermarkets, and Asian groceries.

Asian ginseng can be overstimulating, however. The symptoms of overstimulation include a stiff neck and headache. If these symptoms occur while taking Asian ginseng, stop taking it, and try a different remedy.

rather than an indication of mental illness. If you decide to participate in therapy, it's important that you find a counselor who's right for you. In a counseling situation, you should feel safe—physically and emotionally. Keep in mind you are investing your money, time, and effort, and no therapist, no matter how skilled, works well with all clients. The goal is to find the right fit between your personality and problems and the therapist's personality and expertise.

Many personal emotional problems can be greatly improved or even permanently overcome within six visits to a psychotherapist. The therapist often then becomes an ally that the individual can visit occasionally during crises or periods of change.

☞ DIRECTIONS: Ask a friend for a referral, or consult a directory of local therapists. Talk to a few therapists on the phone or in person before making a selection. Explain what you need help with and ask candidates if they've had any experience in this area. Try to determine which therapist you feel a "chemistry" with. Also, ask about the therapist's training and qualifications.

Beating Depression

According to *Herbal Medicine Past and Present* (Volume I), by John K. Crellin and Jane Philpott, there is plenty of non-herbal advice for the depressed patient. Suggested methods for overcoming depression include paying attention to diet, spending time in the fresh air, exercising, taking a break in routine, getting away from it all, engaging in amusements, being in nature, and working on discovering why you're depressed.

BLACK COHOSH: The American Indians used black cohosh *(Cimicifuga racemosa)* to treat menstrual complaints. Later, the Eclectic physicians adopted the plant, and it soon became one of the most commonly prescribed herbs for treating depression, especially depression associated with the menstrual cycle. Today, black cohosh is an approved antidepressant in Germany.

☞ DIRECTIONS: Purchase a tincture of black cohosh in a health food store or herb shop. Take 1 dropperful three times a day for up to three months, taking breaks during the menstrual period. Also, you can purchase a standardized extract of black cohosh at a health food store and take it as directed.

BONESET: Boneset *(Eupatorium perfoliatum)*, taken as a cold tea, was a famous remedy for sluggish liver (see sidebar, "The Sluggish Liver," on page 146) and melancholy in the colonies before American independence. Previously, boneset was used as a witchcraft medicine by the Iroquois Indians. Cold boneset tea is bitter, which stimulates digestive secretions and bile production by the liver.

☞ DIRECTIONS: Put 1 teaspoon of dried boneset leaves in a cup. Fill the cup with boiling water, and let the tea stand until it is room temperature. Drink one third of the cup before meals, three times a day, for a week or two.

❧ Diarrhea ❧

❖ ❖ ❖

Diarrhea is abnormally frequent and excessively liquid bowel movements. This is often the body's defensive attempt to rid itself of irritating or toxic substances. It is a symptom that accompanies many disorders, both mild and serious.

There are two basic types of diarrhea: acute (or short-term) diarrhea, the more common form, which comes on quickly and usually lasts no more than two or three days, although it can last as long as two weeks; and chronic (or long-term) diarrhea, which may also appear suddenly but lingers for many weeks or months, with symptoms either constantly present or appearing and disappearing.

Both acute and chronic diarrhea can become a serious problem because of the excessive loss of body fluids (called dehydration) and the loss of the nutrients sodium, potassium, and chloride. Simply drinking more water is not sufficient to replace these losses. Minerals as well as glucose must be replaced in severe diarrhea. Electrolyte replacement drinks for infants are readily available in grocery stores. Use of such replacement liquids has revolutionized diarrhea care for infants throughout the Third World in the last ten years, where diarrhea is a leading cause of infant death. The accompanying sidebar shows the composition of electrolyte replacement formulas (see sidebar, "Electrolyte Replacement Therapy," page 158).

In an infection, the intestines may pour out massive quantities of fluids and salts in response to a bacterial toxin (poison) or other irritant. Viruses may cause minor epidemics of diarrhea, usually referred to as "intestinal flu." (The influenza virus is actually not involved.) In inflammatory bowel disease (also known as colitis), protein, blood, and mucus are lost through the inflamed lining of the colon; large quantities of water are also lost. Other disorders speed up the normal movement of the colon, thereby not allowing time for absorption of fluids. Yet another type of diarrhea is caused by poor absorption of a type of sugar (called lactose) that draws fluid out of the colon. Other causes of diarrhea include changes in the diet, certain medications, stress, and food allergies. Diarrhea is a symptom and not a disease, and conventional treatment for diarrhea varies widely depending on the cause. Most important is the replacement of fluids and electrolytes if diarrhea is severe. Constipating drugs or bulk fiber may also be given. Common medical wisdom, both conventional and alternative, is to let normal mild diarrhea run its course because it is a natural defense mechanism that washes infectious bacteria, viruses, or toxins out of the body. Diarrhea may be suppressed with constipating astringents, whether herbal or over-the-counter, but that may make you sicker. According to *My Water Cure,* by Father

Sebastian Kneipp, a 19th century German peasant priest and folk healer: "Sudden stopping of diarrhea is never to be recommended: the foul matters should be gradually removed...."

The folk remedies below focus on removing or correcting the cause of the condition.

Remedies

BLACKBERRY ROOT: Perhaps the most commonly recommended remedy for diarrhea in North American folklore is blackberry root tea. Blackberry roots *(Rubus hispidus)* are not usually available in the commercial herb trade, but, if you are willing to brave the thorns, then start picking—the plant grows throughout most of the United States.

Taking blackberry root was a popular remedy in the United States during the 1800s. A listing in the 1849 book *The Family Physician* states that

Kitchen Spices for Diarrhea

Many folk remedies for diarrhea use simple kitchen spices. These spices are probably most appropriate for treating simple diarrhea that results from poor digestion and malabsorption, not severe diarrhea that's caused by an infectious agent. The volatile oils in the spices may also be effective against mild intestinal "flu." The oils act as digestive stimulants, increasing the natural digestive secretions of the stomach, intestines, and gallbladder. Because the stomach acid and digestive enzymes can destroy some invading organisms, the oils may have an indirect effect against infectious organisms. The kitchen spices basil, cinnamon, clove, ginger, nutmeg, black pepper, cayenne pepper, and thyme have all been mentioned in North American folk tradition as treatments for diarrhea.

Electrolyte Replacement Therapy

The World Health Organization recommends the following formula for electrolyte replacement after excessive diarrhea or vomiting:

3.5 grams sodium chloride (table salt)

2.5 grams sodium bicarbonate (baking soda)

1.5 grams potassium chloride (available at a pharmacy)

20 grams of glucose (available at a pharmacy)

Add the ingredients to a liter (1 quart, 2 ounces) of water and drink.

For electrolyte replacement, you can also try the formula below. This remedy, taken from a German medical text, includes peppermint, which is a traditional folk treatment for diarrhea.

☞ DIRECTIONS: Make a tea by simmering 1 tablespoon each of peppermint leaves and fennel seed in 1 quart of water for fifteen minutes in a covered pot. Strain and allow to cool to room temperature. Add ¹/₂ teaspoon salt, ¹/₄ teaspoon baking soda, ¹/₄ teaspoon potassium chloride, and 2 tablespoons glucose. Drink freely.

blackberry root "often provides a sovereign remedy [for diarrhea] when all other remedies fail." The text states that, during a dysentery epidemic, none of the local Indians using blackberry root died, while many of their white neighbors did. The root was used to treat diarrhea by the Oneida, Rappahannock, and Shinnecock Indians. It was likely that the whites died of mercury poisoning—mercury was what the white physicians used to treat diarrhea at the time.

The use of blackberry root for treating diarrhea survives today in the folk medicine of New England, Indiana, Appalachia, and among the Amish in the eastern states. The roots contain astringent tannins, which dry up the watery secretions of the intestines. The following suggestion comes from the folk traditions of New England.

☞ DIRECTIONS: Simmer a handful of the roots in 1 pint of water until the liquid turns dark. Drink 1 cup. Wait a few hours and, if necessary, drink another. Don't take more than 2 cups a day. Gather the roots in the fall.

WORMWOOD: German immigrants at the turn of the century used wormwood tincture *(Artemisia absinthium)* to treat diarrhea. They arrived in this country carrying with them a popular health book called *My Water Cure* (English translation) by Father Sebastian Kneipp. The book warned against taking the remedy for a prolonged period of time or at high doses.

In the past, Europeans who consumed large amounts of wormwood, via an alcoholic drink called absinthe, developed a form of insanity. The artist Vincent Van Gogh probably suffered from this mental illness, which may account for his progressive insanity and the increasing hallucinatory quality of his paintings at the end of his life.

A related plant from New Mexico, estafiate *(Artemisa ludoviciana),* is used identically in the folk medicine there. New Mexican folklorist Michael Moore suggests that wormwood treats minor diarrhea by restoring normal secretions of the stomach acid and bile.

☞ DIRECTIONS: Purchase a tincture of wormwood in a health food store. Take a dropperful three times a day for no more than two days for treating simple diarrhea.

CHARCOAL: The use of charcoal for treating diarrhea in North America was well under way before the arrival of the European colonists. The Kwakiutl tribe from the Pacific Northwest would burn the bark of a fir tree, pulverize the coals, add the ash to water (sometimes with other herbs), and drink the mixture to end diarrhea. The use of "hardwood ashes" in water to treat diarrhea is also recorded by folklorist Clarence Meyer in his folk collection *American Folk Medicine.* Today, the use of charcoal to treat diarrhea is used by the Amish and Seventh Day Adventists.

Charcoal is absorbent, meaning that toxic substances attach to it and are tightly bound. It is used in emergency medicine to treat some types of poisoning. Be sure to use activated charcoal, which is very finely powdered and treated to be free of contaminants and gases.

☞ DIRECTIONS: Purchase charcoal capsules from a pharmacy. Take 4 to 8 capsules three to four times a day.

ORANGE PEEL TEA: In reference to orange peel, a 9th century medical text from Baghdad, Iraq, says that "candied skin"

is good for the stomach. Orange peel teas were used to treat digestive problems in Arabic medicine and European medicine during the Middle Ages, until the 1600s. The peels of related citrus fruits are still used for treating digestive complaints in China and India today. The practice also survives in the folklore of Indiana.

The oils in the peels stimulate digestion. (Today, dyes and pesticides are used on oranges, so if you want to try this remedy, you'll have to obtain organic oranges.) An Indiana remedy says to drink freely of orange peel tea sweetened with sugar.

☞ DIRECTIONS: Peel 1 organic orange and chop the skin into small pieces. Place the skin in a pot and cover with 1 pint of boiling water. Cover well and let stand until the water reaches room temperature. Sweeten with sugar or honey and drink freely.

CHAMOMILE (GERMAN): German immigrants to the United States used German chamomile *(Matricaria recutita)* to treat diarrhea. Chamomile is also mentioned as a treatment for diarrhea in Gypsy folklore.

Chamomile contains strong anti-inflammatory oils as well as other active principles. It may be best used in treating diarrhea caused by intestinal inflammation. Modern studies show it has anti-spasmodic properties as well. One German source suggests combining the tea half-and-half with peppermint. A Gypsy treatment calls for adding 25 blueberries to the tea. Thus, chamomile is probably viewed in folk medicine as a supportive treatment rather than a singular one. The following suggestion offers contemporary German advice.

☞ DIRECTIONS: Place 1 teaspoon of chamomile flowers and 1 teaspoon of peppermint leaves in a cup. Fill with boiling water. Let steep, covered, for fifteen minutes. Sweeten, if desired, and drink 3 cups a day.

❧ Digistion ❧

▦ ▦ ▦

If the digestive tract is healthy and digestion and absorption of the nutrients are efficient, then the entire body will be well nourished and will function optimally. Any irregularity in digestion, however, can cause or contribute to disease anywhere in the body.

Below are some common signs of a poorly functioning digestive system:

- flatulence or belching
- nausea
- pain anywhere in the digestive tract
- undigested food in the stool
- offensive breath
- constipation (less than one bowel movement per day)
- lethargy after meals
- food cravings other than normal hunger
- lack of satisfaction after meals
- lack of hunger for breakfast

These symptoms—all considered to be serious signs that require treatment in traditional medical systems—are often left untreated by conventional physicians in North America. This is not so in the modern medicine of Germany and France, however, where symptoms such as "biliousness" (sluggish liver function), poor appetite, gas, and bloating or feelings of fullness after meals are routinely treated by doctors, often with herbal medicines from the European folk tradition.

According to folk medicine throughout the world, which offers many remedies for weak and sluggish digestion, healthy digestion requires:

- a balance of fats, proteins, and starches in the diet, and adequate fiber from sources such as fruits and vegetables.

■ food intake in moderate quantities. Overeating strains the capacity of the digestive system to process the consumed food, and undigested or partially digested remnants can cause inflammation and other problems in the digestive tract and elsewhere in the body.

■ a relaxed state during meals. For the stomach and intestines to function normally, and for digestive secretions to be adequate, the body cannot be in a state of stress during meals.

■ a healthy number of normal bacteria in the gut. The "garden" of friendly bacteria in the intestines acts as a defense against harmful bacteria, yeasts, molds, and other micro-organisms by competing with them for food. (As the friendly bacteria proliferate, the nutrients they consume deprive the harmful microorganisms of their food supply.) Some of these friendly bacteria manufacture essential vitamins. The good bacteria can be disrupted by courses of such drugs as birth control pills, steroids, and antibiotics, however, leading to poor digestion and inflammation and infection of the intestinal wall. This in turn can cause inflammatory diseases in other parts of the body as the intestinal contents leak through the inflamed gut wall and overwhelm the immune system.

Folk remedies may improve digestion by stimulating the secretion of more stomach acid, digestive enzymes, and bile (a digestive secretion of the liver) from the liver. The remedies may also improve the absorption of nutrients by increasing blood flow to the mucous membranes of the intestines. Finally, antispasmodic constituents in folk remedies may prevent spasms in intestinal wall muscles that often accompany gas and bloating. Any severe or persistent digestive tract symptoms merit a visit to a doctor, however.

Remedies

GINGER: Ginger (*Zingiber officinale*) is a folk remedy for treating gas or nausea in the folk traditions of both New England and the southern Appalachians. It is used the same way in the traditional medicine of India, China, and Arabia. Ginger contains at least 13 antispasmodic constituents, which may help reduce spasms and tension in the digestive tract muscles. Also, circulatory stimulants in ginger increase circulation to the mucous membrane lining of the digestive tract, which in turn increases digestive secretions and absorption of nutrients. What's more, in clinical trials, ginger has shown to be effective in soothing some kinds of nausea and vertigo. Avoid excessive doses of ginger if you're taking drugs for heart or blood conditions or diabetes.

☞ DIRECTIONS: Stir ½ teaspoon of ground ginger into a cup of hot water. Let stand two to three minutes. Strain and drink.

MINTS: Different types of mints are recommended for treating indigestion in North American folk literature, most commonly peppermint (*Mentha piperita*) and spearmint (*Mentha spicata*). Mints appear in the folk medicine of New England, New York, Indiana, Appalachia, New Mexico, and California. Mints have also been used as carminatives (see sidebar, page 168) by members of the Cherokee, Chippewa, Dakota, Omaha, Pawnee, Ponca, and Winnebago American Indian tribes. Mint species contain the antispasmodic constituents carvacrol, eugenol, limonene, and thymol, which may help reduce intestinal spasms. A contemporary German medical text, *Lehrbuch der Phytotherapie* by R. F. Weiss, M.D. (in translation: *Herbal Medicine*), recommends the mints as digestive aids for their carminative and antispasmodic

Bitter Tonics

In folk medicine and traditional herbalism, bitter tonics are one of the most often prescribed categories of herbs and foods. In fact, a 1994 poll of the most-often prescribed medicinal herbs by North American professional herbalists showed that half of the top ten herbs had important bitter constituents.

The key indication for bitter tonics is poor appetite. The bitter constituents in the plants stimulate the secretion of stomach acid and liver bile, thereby improving digestion and nourishment. Because they stimulate these secretions, however, they are contraindicated if you have heartburn or other kinds of digestive pain.

Bitter tonics in this section include wormwood, chamomile, goldenseal, Oregon grape root, gentian, and boneset. Bitter tonics are often combined with carminative herbs in simple formulas (see sidebar, "Carminatives," page 168).

properties. Peppermint is used as an official digestive aid in Germany.

☞ DIRECTIONS: Place 1 teaspoon of the dried herb in a cup and add boiling water. Cover and let stand for ten minutes. Strain well and drink the tea warm three times a day on an empty stomach. Don't take peppermint if you are experiencing heartburn or painful belching.

FENNEL: A tea of fennel seeds *(Foeniculum vulgare)* is used for treating sluggish digestion or gas in the folk medicine of both New England and China. It is also the most often prescribed tea for abdominal cramping and gas in adults in the medical herbalism of contemporary Great Britain, Canada, and the United States. It is an approved medicine in Germany for mild gastrointestinal complaints. At least 16 chemical constituents in fennel have demonstrated antispasmodic effects in animal trials.

☞ DIRECTIONS: Place 1 teaspoon of the seeds in a cup and add boiling water. Cover and let stand for ten minutes. Strain well and drink three cups of warm tea a day on an empty stomach until digestion improves.

CARAWAY SEEDS: Caraway seeds *(Carum carvi),* with a flavor and a medicinal action similar to that of fennel are recommended for gas and poor digestion in Appalachia and in the folk medicine of Indiana. Their medicinal use originated in Arab culture. Their use for poor digestion spread to ancient Rome, and from there to European folk medicine. Caraway seeds are approved for medical use for weak digestion by the German government.

☞ DIRECTIONS: In a cup, pour boiling water over 1 teaspoon of the crushed seeds. Cover and let stand for ten minutes. Strain well and drink three cups of warm tea a day on an empty stomach.

Alternately, you can chew on the seeds. A common practice in households in India and the Middle East is to pass a small bowl of caraway, fennel, or anise seeds for nibbling after meals.

AMERICAN GINSENG: American ginseng *(Panax quinquefolium)* is used as a digestive tonic throughout the Appalachian mountain chain where it grows. A related species of ginseng *(Panax ginseng),* known as Asian ginseng, is perhaps the most famous tonic herb in China. (American ginseng, however, is also exported to China in large quantities.)

Even though both species are called "ginseng," the Chinese use the two plants for entirely different purposes. Asian ginseng is considered to be stimulating; in fact, it is sometimes used in large doses as a stimulant in Chinese hospital emergency rooms. American ginseng, however, is used as a sedative for individuals who are tense and nervous from prolonged stress or illness.

American ginseng earned the attention of the turn-of-the-century medical doctor Arthur Harding, M.D., who, out of disillusionment with the conventional medicines of his day, abandoned his regular medical practice in order to investigate folk remedies. He said in his book *Ginseng and Other Medicinal Plants*, published in 1909: "If the people of the United States were educated as to its use, our supply of ginseng would be consumed in our own country and it would be a hard blow to the medical profession." In his book, Harding recounts case studies of patients whose generally deteriorated health improved only after a few weeks or months of treatment with ginseng. He attributes the plant's power to restore health to its ability to restore weak digestion.

Unlike Asian ginseng, very little scientific research has been performed on American ginseng. Thus, we have to rely on contemporary Chinese medicine or on the folk traditions of this country for guidance on its use.

☞ DIRECTIONS: American ginseng can cost more than $200 a pound, and many adulterated products are sold in health food stores. The most reliable way to use it is to make your own powder from whole roots with the fine rootlets attached.

Purchase the roots and grind them into powder in a coffee grinder. (Consume the powder from one root before grinding another, because the constituents are more likely to be preserved in the whole root than in the powder.) Stir ¼ to ½ teaspoon of the powder into 1 cup of warm water and drink one dose daily on an empty stomach before breakfast for two to three weeks. Then, repeat if desired after taking a break for one or two weeks.

Carminatives

Carminative herbs and spices are hot digestive stimulants that have traditionally been taken for indigestion accompanied by gas. Exactly how they work is not clear, but some scientific experiments give us a hint.

German researchers observed that carminative spices may reduce gas pressure in the stomach by promoting belching and the release of gas. Carminatives also increase circulation to the stomach wall, which reduces spasm and improves the absorption of nutrients.

In addition, according to a German textbook on medical herbalism called *Lehrbuch der Phytotherapie* by R. F. Weiss, M.D. (translation: *Herbal Medicine*), which is used in schools of medicine and pharmacy in Germany, carminatives improve the tone of the intestinal muscles and increase the secretion of digestive juices. These herbs and spices invariably contain antispasmodic substances as well, which is why a key indication for using carminatives is poor digestion accompanied by gas or spasm. Carminatives are often combined with bitter herbs in formulas.

CHAMOMILE (GERMAN): Chamomile *(Matricaria recutita)* is recommended for intestinal spasm or gas in the folk traditions of New England, Indiana, and the American Southwest. It combines both antispasmodic and sedative properties and may relieve intestinal cramping and induce relaxation at the same time. Chamomile contains at least 19 antispasmodic constituents, as well as five sedative ones. The plant is approved in Germany as a medicine for gastrointestinal complaints. In addition, a 1993 clinical trial in Germany showed that chamomile was effective in relieving colic.

continued on page 170

Worms Be Gone!

■ ■ ■

In folk medicine, from aloe to yucca root, the catalog of plant-based remedies for worms is long. The most widely used medicine in the country for a century and a half was the Cherokee recipe for pulverized root of pinkroot. Plant-based teas used across the country included pumpkin seed, horsemint, peach leaf, and butternut bark. Garlic was a mainstay, usually eaten but sometimes worn on a string around the neck. Recommended foods included burnt toast, sauerkraut, and raw potatoes.

If these remedies didn't work, people could try patent medicines, whose makers were quick to exploit the grotesque potential of worms. Medicine-show men displayed roundworms in jars for their customers' contemplation.

The ancient theory that something repulsive must be driven out by something even worse is evident in worm remedies with appalling ingredients, such as tea of earthworm, sulphur, or kerosene. One of the most common "cures" was also the most dangerous: turpentine.

Perhaps it was a good thing that there were magical cures as well. Some charms addressed the worms themselves. One from 13th century England begins, "I adjure you, worms, in the name . . . ." It may be compared with one recorded in Pennsylvania six hundred years later: "Worm, I conjure thee by the living God that thou avoid this flesh and blood."

The belief that a tapeworm eats the "host's" food inspired the Scottish cure whereby the sufferer chews bread, spits it out, then drinks some whiskey. The worms smell the bread, open their mouths, and are choked by the alcohol. No longer an everyday worry, worms still wiggle into our folklore.

☞ DIRECTIONS: Pour boiling water over 1 tablespoon of chamomile flowers in a cup. Cover and let sit for ten minutes. Strain and drink warm three times a day on an empty stomach. Do this for two to three weeks. Taking one of the doses before bed may also work as a sleep aid. Avoid using if signs of allergy appear. Avoid excessive use during pregnancy and lactation.

WORMWOOD: Wormwood (*Artemisia absinthium, Artemisia spp.*) is described as a digestive stimulant in the Hispanic folk medicine of southern California. The active constituents of wormwood include bitter digestive stimulants and anti-inflammatory volatile oils including azulenes, constituents that are also present in chamomile. The European species of the plant is approved as a digestive stimulant by the German government.

☞ DIRECTIONS: Place 1 teaspoon of wormwood leaves in a cup of water and fill with boiling water. Cover well to prevent the escape of aromatic substances. Let cool to room temperature. Take ½ doses three or four times a day. Don't take wormwood for more than ten days at a time and take a ten-day break before starting the therapy again. Avoid excessive consumption.

CINNAMON: Cinnamon (*Cinnamomum verum*) is used as a digestive stimulant in the folk medicine of New England and China. It is also used for this purpose in the Hispanic folk medicine of the Southwest. Cinnamon contains at least 16 different antispasmodic constituents, especially in its aromatic oils. It contains the antispasmodic and circulatory stimulant cinnamaldehyde in large quantities. Cinnamon is approved by the German government for treatment of poor digestion. It is contraindicated in medicinal quantities during pregnancy, however, because it can stimulate uterine contractions.

☞ DIRECTIONS: Stir ¼ to ½ teaspoon of cinnamon powder into a cup of hot water. Let stand three to five minutes. Stir again and drink without straining.

GENTIAN: In this country, five of the six North American gentian species were used as digestive aids or bitter tonics by American Indians. Gentian *(Gentiana lutea)* is the most famous component of the pre-dinner "bitters" commonly consumed in European folk medicine. (Bitters are traditionally taken in many cultures ten to twenty minutes before meals to improve the appetite.) Experiments show that bitters increase the secretion of stomach acid, which helps the digestive system prepare for the meal.

The use of gentian also appears in the contemporary folk literature of British Columbia. Gentian is approved as a bitter tonic by the German government. Like other strong bitters, it is contraindicated if you are experiencing heartburn or other digestive pain or if you have an ulcer.

☞ DIRECTIONS: Chop up three fresh lemon peels and place with 1 ounce of chopped gentian root in 1 quart of water. Bring to a boil and simmer on the lowest heat for ten minutes. Let stand until the tea reaches room temperature. Strain and store in the refrigerator. Take a teaspoon twenty minutes before meals. If the gentian causes heartburn, stop taking it. Avoid in pregnancy and lactation.

GOLDENSEAL AND OREGON GRAPE ROOT: Goldenseal *(Hydrastis canadensis)* is the most famous bitter tonic in North American folk medicine. The colonists learned its use from the American Indians, and it entered into the folk medicine of New England in the 1700s. Goldenseal remained a common household remedy throughout the eastern states during the 1800s. It was also one of the most commonly pre-

Fiber and Digestion

German naturopathic tradition, which arrived in this country with turn-of-the-century German immigrants, has long advocated a high fiber diet to improve poor digestion. In the last 20 years, conventional medicine has begun to recommend the same.

What is the single most important dietary change you can make to improve digestion? Eat more fiber, and not as fiber supplements, but in the form of whole foods—grains, beans, fruits, and vegetables. Fiber provides bulk for the stool, helping to maintain muscle tone in the intestinal walls. The result is faster passage of food through the intestines and less constipation. Fiber also feeds the friendly bacteria in the digestive tract, increasing their number and creating a defense against potentially harmful bacteria.

scribed herbs by doctors of the Eclectic and Physiomedicalist schools of medicine. Although goldenseal had several therapeutic uses, the physicians often prescribed it to restore the functioning of a "run-down" digestive system.

Today, goldenseal is an endangered species, so medical herbalists in North America frequently prescribe Oregon grape root (*Mahonia aquifolium, Berberis aquifolium*) as a substitute bitter tonic. (Because of its equivalent bitter effects, Eclectic physicians also prescribed Oregon grape root.) As with other strong bitters, don't take either of these herbs if you are experiencing digestive pain or if you have an ulcer.

☞ DIRECTIONS: Grind Oregon grape root in a coffee grinder to make a powder. Stir ½ teaspoon into a cup of hot water. Allow to stand for three to five minutes. Don't strain, just stir. Drink the cup twenty minutes before meals for one to three weeks.

BONESET: Contemporary North Carolina folk traditions suggest taking a tea of boneset *(Eupatorium perfoliatum)* for weak digestion. Boneset was one of the most common folk remedies in the early American colonies, where it was considered to be a panacea. It was taken as a hot tea to treat colds, flu, and feverish diseases. As a cold tea, it was used as a bitter digestive tonic. Boneset is very bitter to the taste.

☞ DIRECTIONS: Place 1 tablespoon of dried boneset leaves in a 1-pint jar and fill with boiling water. Cover and let cool to room temperature. Drink half of a cup twenty minutes before meals for one to three weeks.

CATNIP: Catnip *(Nepeta cataria)* tea, a sedative and indigestion remedy in European folk medicine, has been a popular remedy in this country since the arrival of the European immigrants. The plant rapidly became naturalized here, and American Indian tribes such as the Onondaga and Cayuga eventually used it for poor digestion as well, especially when treating children. It was an official medicine in the *United States Pharmacopoeia* from 1840 until 1870.

Catnip has been used in folk medicine to treat weak digestion, intestinal spasm, and gas by residents of New England, Appalachia, North Carolina, Indiana, and New Mexico and by Blacks throughout the deep South and by Chicanos in Los Angeles. Catnip combines both carminative and sedative properties, with seven antispasmodic and five sedative constituents.

☞ DIRECTIONS: Pour boiling water over 1 teaspoon of the dried herb. Let sit covered for ten minutes. Strain and drink three cups a day, between meals on an empty stomach.

WATER TREATMENT: A treatment for weak digestion, gas, and bloating from the Seventh Day Adventists tradition is to apply a heating pad or hot water bottle to the abdomen after meals. This presumably attracts circulation to the area, improving digestion. Relaxation during the period of application also promotes good digestion.

☞ DIRECTIONS: Place a hot water bottle or heating pad over the abdomen and relax, lying down, for twenty minutes after meals.

CASTOR OIL: A suggestion for poor digestion, from the folk medicine of contemporary Indiana, is to apply a warm castor oil pack to the abdomen. Castor oil taken internally is a strong laxative. It does not have this effect with external applications, however.

The external use of castor oil for digestive pain and complaints gained popularity in North American folk traditions in the second half of the 20th century, thanks to the advice of mystic Edgar Cayce, who was known for giving medical advice while in a trance-like state. His books on health remain popular throughout the United States today.

Cayce claimed that castor oil packs improved the functioning of the gut's immune system. No scientific evidence exists to support this claim, although the practice appears to be harmless. Some benefits from the treatment may come from the relaxation and hot application involved. Castor oil packs for digestive problems are now a standard treatment in North American naturopathic medicine.

☞ DIRECTIONS: Dip a cloth in castor oil and apply to the abdomen. Cover with plastic wrap and a second cloth, and finally with a heating pad on low heat. (The plastic wrap keeps the castor oil away from the heating pad.) Relax with the pad in place for forty to sixty minutes in the evening after dinner three nights a week. Do not use if appendicitis is suspected or during pregnancy.

❧ Eczema ❧

❑ ❑ ❑

Eczema is an inflammation of the skin and is most commonly equated with the medical term atopic dermatitis. It is characterized by red, oozing, and sometimes crusty lesions on the face, the scalp, the extremities, and the diaper area in infants. The lesions may also become infected with bacteria or other microorganisms, and infection with herpes virus can cause serious illness. Stress, food allergens, scratching, bathing, and sweating may also induce attacks.

Conventional treatment includes avoidance of triggers and administration of antihistamine topical steroid creams and antibiotics for infections of the eczema lesions. Alternative medical treatments include avoidance of triggers; optimizing vitamin, mineral, and essential fatty acid nutrition to reduce tendency to develop inflammation; internal or topical applications of anti-inflammatory or soothing herbs; and administration of bitter herbs to "stimulate the liver" and optimize digestion.

In alternative medicine, it is believed that to heal the skin, you must heal the digestive tract as well.

Thus, a three-way link that exists between the liver, the digestive tract, and the skin is a key tenet of alternative medicine for treating allergic eczema and other skin inflammations. One physiological basis for this theory may be the detoxifying role of the liver. The liver normally transforms toxic substances so they can be excreted from the body either in the form of bile from the liver or as urine. If the liver is not doing its job, toxic substances may circulate freely in the body and irritate the skin "from the inside out."

The folk treatments below include bitter herbs to stimulate the liver and digestive tract, anti-inflammatory herbs for both internal and external use, astringent and disinfectant herbs for topical use, and treatments with water and clay.

Remedies

NETTLE AND DANDELION: A Gypsy folk remedy for eczema uses a combination of two "blood purifying" herbs (see "Blood Purifiers and Blood Builders," page 79) that are traditionally prescribed to treat skin conditions. Stinging nettle *(Urtica dioica, U. urens)* has been used by at least seven American Indian tribes—from the northeastern United States to the Pacific Northwest and down to Mexico—as an aid for healing skin conditions. Stinging nettle is used for the same purpose in traditional European herbalism. A recent clinical trial showed that nettle was effective for treating hay fever, and recent laboratory research has identified its anti-inflammatory and anti-allergic constituents.

Dandelion root is traditionally considered to be a "liver" herb—its use in this country is consistent with the traditional idea of treating skin ailments through the liver (see introduction to this section, above). It has been used to treat skin conditions by several American Indian tribes, including the

Iroquois of the northeastern United States, the Aleuts of the Pacific Northwest, and the Tewa of the Southwest. The German government has approved the medicinal use of dandelion root as a "cholagogue," a medicine that increases the flow of bile from the liver.

Constituents in dandelion have also been found to protect the liver and to enhance its detoxifying ability. Dandelion contains both antioxidant and anti-inflammatory constituents.

☞ DIRECTIONS: Place 1 ounce of dandelion root and 1 ounce of nettle leaf in a pot, and cover with 3 pints of water. Bring to a boil and then simmer, covered, on low heat for forty minutes. Let cool to room temperature. Drink 3 cups a day. Do this for three weeks, and then take a break for seven to ten days before starting again.

BURDOCK ROOT: In the traditional herbalism of Europe and North America, burdock (*Arctium lappa, A. minus*) is probably the most well-known for treating skin complaints such as acne, boils, or eczema. It has been used to treat skin conditions by several American Indian tribes, including the Cherokee, Iroquois, Menominee, Micmac, Nanticoke, and Penobscot. Burdock is used today in folk medicine as a "blood purifier" among Pennsylvania Germans, the Amish, Indiana farmers, and throughout Appalachia. Burdock was an official medicine in the *United States Pharmacopoeia* from 1831 until 1842, and again from 1851 until 1916; it was prescribed as a diuretic, mild laxative, and treatment for skin ailments.

Modern scientific studies show that constituents in burdock root have anti-inflammatory properties. Its constituent poly- saccharide inulin, which can make up 50 percent of the root by weight, provides food for the "friendly" strains of bacteria in the gut and may thus help reduce the toxic load on the liver and skin by reducing toxicity in the bowels.

For some individuals, however, burdock can worsen eczema. Perhaps this is because burdock promotes light sweating, and sweat can trigger eczema in some people. If you find that burdock makes your eczema worse, stop using it immediately and try a different remedy.

☞ DIRECTIONS: Put 1 ounce of burdock root in 1 quart of water. Bring the water to a boil and simmer, covered, for forty minutes. Drink the quart throughout the day. Burdock is a mild herb and can be consumed this way for long periods of time.

YELLOW DOCK: Yellow dock (*Rumex crispus*), like dandelion and burdock, is a traditional bitter, liver-stimulating herb. The Aleut, Cherokee, Cheyenne, Iroquois, Navaho, and Shoshone Indians, as well as other American Indian tribes, used it to treat skin ailments. It was a folk remedy for treating eczema of residents of the eastern states in the 1800s. It was listed in the *United States Pharmacopoeia* from 1860 until 1890; physicians of the last century used it to treat chronic skin ailments. It is still used today for this purpose in the Southwest.

☞ DIRECTIONS: Make a tincture of yellow dock by placing 4 ounces of the dried root in a 1-quart jar and filling the jar with 100 proof vodka or gin. Let stand for three weeks, shaking the jar once a day. Strain and store in a cool dark place. The dose is 2 to 3 droppers twice a day, taken in a cup of warm water. Alternately, you can purchase a tincture of yellow dock at a health food or herb store.

HONEY: Honey is a traditional remedy for infected eczema throughout Asia. Honey is also used by Chinese Americans. Honey is a powerful disinfectant and has been used by conventional physicians in both France and India as a disinfectant for burns.

☞ DIRECTIONS: Cover gauze with a layer of honey, place over the eczema, and cover with tape or a bandage. Change the dressing every two hours until the infection is gone.

BAKING SODA BATH: Contemporary Seventh Day Adventists recommend treating eczema by taking a baking soda bath. In New England, the same treatment is used for relieving hives and other skin conditions.

☞ DIRECTIONS: Place a few handfuls of baking soda in warm bath water and take a long soak.

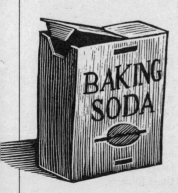

YARROW: Yarrow (*Achillea spp.*) is used as a universal treatment for skin ailments (including infected wounds) by the American Indians. In fact, a database of American Indian ethnobotany at the University of Michigan records the use of yarrow by 24 tribes for remedying skin conditions.

Yarrow contains the constituents azulene and chamazulene, both of which are antiallergic and anti-inflammatory. A strong tea of yarrow has been found to be more effective than steroid creams to suppress eczema. As with steroid creams, however, as soon as the treatment is stopped, the eczema returns. Thus, internal remedies as well as identification and removal of triggers are important for long-term healing.

☞ DIRECTIONS: Place 1 ounce of yarrow leaves in a 1-quart canning jar and fill with boiling water. Cover tightly to prevent the active constituents from escaping with the steam. Let cool to room temperature. Apply with gauze to the eczema three or four times a day.

CHAMOMILE: Today, residents of Mexico and the American Southwest use a wash of chamomile tea *(Matricaria recutita)* to treat skin infections. The Cherokee Indians used chamomile to remedy afflictions of the skin as well.

For some individuals who are allergic to chamo-mile itself, however, chamomile can cause an allergic skin rash. If you are allergic to it, try using yarrow instead, which contains the same key constituents but belongs to another plant family and is not as likely to provoke an allergic response.

☞ DIRECTIONS: Place 1 teaspoon of chamomile flowers in a cup and fill with boiling water. Cover and let stand for ten minutes. Strain well, cool, then apply several times a day.

❧ Fatigue ❧

Fatigue may be physical or mental exhaustion, an overwhelming feeling of weariness, or a lack of energy and enthusiasm for even pleasant activities. Fatigue is a symptom of a vast number of diseases and disorders. More than 10 million people visit their doctors each year complaining of fatigue, making fatigue the seventh most common reason we make a doctor's appointment. Between one-fourth and one-fifth of all Americans will seek medical advice for severe or chronic fatigue at some point in their lives.

The remedies in this section are appropriate for treating normal, brief periods of fatigue that are the result of some unusual stress or unexpected disruption of sleep. Any severe or long-lasting fatigue requires a medical checkup to determine the cause.

Fatigue and tiring rapidly with minimal activity are often among the early signs of an approaching illness. Fatigue is a warning sign of a variety of diseases and disorders, including the common cold, influenza, hepatitis, infectious mononucleosis, and other infectious diseases; heart disease; lung disorders, such as emphysema; some glandular diseases, such as diabetes; and anemia and nutritional deficiencies. Deficiencies of the minerals magnesium and zinc, the most common mineral deficiencies in the American population (affecting more than half of us), may cause fatigue in some people as well. Deficiencies of chromium, copper, folic acid, manganese, niacin, pantothenic acid, pyridoxine, thiamine, vitamin A, vitamin B_{12}, vitamin C, iron, and potassium may also be responsible. Overwork, either mental or physical, may also cause fatigue, as can psychological disorders or emotional stress. Sugar and caffeine consumption can also result in severe or chronic fatigue in some individuals.

Fatigue is best remedied by treating the physical disorder or psychological problem that is causing it. Some types of fatigue, particularly those due to physical overexertion, can probably be prevented by getting adequate exercise and rest. The average hours of sleep an American gets each night have been on the decline for the last 25 years. We now sleep an average of 7.5 hours a night. That's about an hour less than the average optimal amount of sleep. A third of Americans sleep less than six hours a night; many of them try to catch up by sleeping more on the weekends. A good alternative to sleeping more at night (or on the weekends) is to squeeze in naps during the day. Several folk traditions advocate napping on a regular basis to prevent or treat fatigue.

Remedies

BETONY: A folk source from 1824, listed in folklorist Clarence Meyer's *American Folk Medicine,* states that betony *(Stachys officinalis, Betonica officinalis)* is a good remedy for general debility that arises from disturbed digestion. The original source of this remedy was probably an immigrant from Europe, where betony had been used as a tonic since at least the time of the ancient Romans. In fact, the physician to the Emperor Augustus, who lived at the time of Jesus Christ's birth, listed 47 different diseases he thought betony would cure. The herb has remained so valued in Italy that a popular expression there advises you to "Sell your coat and buy betony."

Although betony is widely used in folk medicine in Europe even today, it has never been used to any extent by North American schools of medicine or by professional herbalists in North America. Betony is the first of the herbs in this section to be classified as a bitter tonic. Betony is also reputed to be a sedative, and its most common use in European herbalism today is for treating nervous tension, nervous headache, and accompanying exhaustion. Don't confuse this plant with North American betony *(Pedicularis spp.),* which grows in the mountainous areas of the West. *Pedicularis,* like *Stachys,* is a sedative, but does not have the bitter tonic properties.

☞ DIRECTIONS: Place 1 tablespoon of betony leaves in a 1-pint jar and fill with boiling water. Cover and let cool until the water reaches room temperature. Drink the pint in 3 doses during the day, twenty minutes before meals, for seven to ten days.

Better Bitter Tonics

In North American herbal traditions, and in the medicine of the 19th century, bitter tonics have been one of the most often prescribed categories of herbs for fatigue and general debility. Bitter tonics are also commonly prescribed for these conditions by conventional physicians in Germany today.

Although these plants possess a mild to strong bitter flavor, they do not have strong medicinal properties. Many act as mild sedatives. The bitter principles in the plants stimulate the secretion of stomach acid and liver bile. Their reputed tonic effects may thus come from improved digestion and nourishment. (Because these herbs stimulate secretions, they are contraindicated if you have heartburn or other kinds of digestive pain.) The most famous of the bitter tonics in North American herbal history are goldthread (*Coptis trifola*), goldenseal (*Hydrastis canadensis*), Oregon grape root (*Mahonia aquifolium, Berberis aquifolium*), yellow dock (*Rumex crispus*), and dandelion root (*Taraxacum officinale*). Goldthread and goldenseal are practically extinct in North America, however. Betony, included in this section, is a common bitter tonic in British herbalism.

OREGON GRAPE ROOT: The American Indians of California and the Pacific Northwest used Oregon grape root *(Mahonia aquifolium, Berberis aquifolium)* to treat general debility. The herb acts as a bitter tonic. Although goldthread *(Coptis trifola)* and goldenseal *(Hydrastis canadensis)* are the most famous of the North American bitter tonics, these herbs have become practically extinct on the continent. Oregon grape root has become the most common substitute for these herbs among North

American professional herbalists. Its action on the digestive system is due to its bitter alkaloid berberine, which is also present in goldthread and goldenseal.

☞ DIRECTIONS: Place 1 tablespoon of Oregon grape root in 1 pint of water. Cover the pot and simmer for twenty minutes. Let cool to room temperature. Drink 1 ounce of the tea twenty minutes before meals for one to three weeks.

NAPPING: The Amish have a saying that a half-hour nap in the afternoon is worth two hours of sleep at night. German immigrants at the turn of the century also advocated the afternoon nap, even if for only fifteen minutes, as an important way to restore energy and prevent exhaustion from overwork.

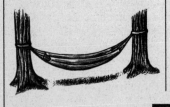

☞ DIRECTIONS: Take a mid-to-late afternoon nap of fifteen minutes or more, lying down if possible.

ASIAN GINSENG: Asian ginseng *(Panax ginseng)* has probably been used in Chinese folk medicine since about 3000 B.C. and remains the most famous and sought after herbal remedy in Chinese culture. In contemporary Chinese medicine, ginseng is used to restore strength when there is physical weakness or exhaustion resulting from a long-term illness. It is also used in folk medicine throughout the modern cities of China, Korea, Japan, and Southeast Asia to increase the individual's ability to resist the stresses of modern life.

Asian ginseng has been used in the folk medicine of Asian communities in North America for at least the last century. In the United States, it entered into mainstream society first through the counter-culture movement of the

1960s and 1970s and then through the health food trade and the current natural healing movement.

Don't take Asian ginseng unless you are run down, because it can be over-stimulating for a person with a normal energy level. Don't take it for chronic fatigue without first getting a thorough medical checkup, because the energy boost from the ginseng may simply temporarily mask the symptoms of a nutritional deficiency or a more serious underlying disease. And don't take ginseng if you also habitually use caffeine. If you begin to experience neck tension, insomnia, increased menstrual flow, or headaches, stop taking ginseng. Prolonged use after experiencing such symptoms can cause high blood pressure.

☞ DIRECTIONS: Purchase a commercial ginseng product in a reputable herb shop. You'll generally find better quality ginseng there than in a health food store, supermarket, or pharmacy. Don't skimp on price—the more expensive products are usually the better quality products. Take 1 to 2 grams of ginseng powder a day, in 2 or 3 doses, for six weeks at a time. Take a two-week break every six weeks.

Also, you can buy some whole ginseng roots—roots of average quality cost about $180 a pound in herb shops. An individual root costs between $6 and $12. Chop 4 ounces of the ginseng root and place in a quart of liquor such as vodka. Cover and let stand for five or six weeks in a cool dark place, turning the jar frequently. Don't strain. Take 1 ounce of the liquid each day, mid-morning or just before lunch.

SIBERIAN GINSENG: Siberian ginseng (*Eleutherococcus senticosus, Acanthopanax senticosus*) has been used in Chinese medicine since the birth of Jesus Christ, but its properties as an adaptogen (see sidebar) were not clearly identified until after World War II. Russian ginseng researchers investigated the Siberian ginseng plant, looking for a less expensive alternative to Asian ginseng. Both animal and human trials showed that the plant increased response and adaptation to stress. The Siberian ginseng preparation remains a popular medicine in Russia today and is available over-the-counter. It is also sometimes prescribed by doctors in Europe.

The term Siberian ginseng was invented by marketers trying to sell the product in the United States in the 1970s, hoping to capitalize on the popularity of Asian ginseng. Siberian ginseng thus entered the folklore of North America through health food stores, and is now widely used in every region of the country. It is important to note that the *Eleutherococcus* plant is not actually a "ginseng," however, and it is nowhere near as powerful as Asian ginseng. But it is also less likely to cause overstimu-lation, insomnia, high blood pressure, or other side effects common to Asian ginseng. Because of its mildness, it is better suited for the average American than is Asian ginseng.

Unfortunately, much of the Siberian ginseng on the market is adulterated. The Canadian government recently examined three shipments arriving from Asia and found that two of them contained no *Eleutherococcus* at all; the other did, but also had 5 percent caffeine added. Most American products are also not made according to the specifications of the Russians and are weak by comparison to the Russian products, sometimes with only one-fifth the strength. For the best products, made according to the specifications of the Russian pharmacopoeia, look for a description such as "1:1 extract in 30% alcohol" on the label of the tincture bottle.

☞ DIRECTIONS: Find a product matching the description above, and take a dropperful of the tincture three times a day for up to six weeks. Take a two-week break before starting another course of treatment.

AN EGG A DAY: Folklorist Clarence Meyer's collection of traditional American remedies called *American Folk Medicine* advises taking an egg a day to restore strength in cases of debility. Deficiencies of several nutrients—including iron, vitamin A, folic acid, riboflavin, and pantothenic acid—may cause fatigue. A single egg contains significant amounts of these nutrients.

☞ DIRECTIONS: Beat a raw egg, flavor with a little sugar or honey, and drink it. If the texture is not appetizing, blend the egg in a glass of milk and drink it that way. Note: Some people caution that a raw egg may be contaminated with salmonella and should be cooked before eating.

❦ Fever ❧

To understand what having a fever means, its helps to know something about how your body controls temperature. There is quite a range in what is considered "normal" in body temperature. (As you know, everyone has a temperature; when it rises above what is considered normal and stays there, it is then termed a fever.) The average human body temperature falls between 98°F and 98.6°F during daily activities, but normal temperatures can range anywhere between 97°F and 99°F. (And many healthy active children have normal temperatures as high as 99°F to 101°F.) Your normal body temperature fluctuates about half a degree during the day, with the lowest reading usually occurring in the early morning and the highest in the late afternoon. The body temperature can be elevated to a range of 101°F to 105°F during fever (or during heavy exercise) and may also fall by about a degree below normal with exposure to cold.

Fever is regulated by a control center in the brain called the hypothalamus. The fever is activated when the hypothalamus senses tiny amounts of bacteria or bacterial toxins in the blood. The hypothalamus may also recognize chemical triggers in the blood that are sent out by white blood cells engaged in fighting off infection.

The hypothalamus is like the thermostat in your house—it is set for a certain temperature range. When it recognizes an infection or immune response, it turns the temperature up. Blood is shunted from the exterior of the body to the interior. As a result, the muscles may involuntarily shiver in order to replace the lost heat. Like a factory suddenly turned up to maximum production, the body's metabolism speeds up by as much as 30 percent in order to produce more white blood cells, antibodies, and other elements of the immune system. Once the infection is successfully fought off, the hypothalamus turns the thermostat back down and the body sweats to cool itself off.

Early in the 20th century, conventional doctors routinely suppressed all fevers with aspirin or related drugs. Modern medicine now recognizes that a fever is a beneficial healing response and mild fevers are no longer routinely suppressed. (Any fever that reaches 104°F or lasts more than three days requires prompt medical attention, however.) The best natural treatment for a simple fever is to support the body's response. Resting in bed, keeping warm, drinking plenty of liquids, and avoiding solid food helps the body to do its job to fight off the infection. Many of the folk remedies below help induce a sweat to cool a fever.

Remedies

GINGER: A fever remedy popular in New England, Appalachia, North Carolina, Indiana, and China is ginger tea. Ginger tea is used to lower fever in the traditional medical systems of India and Arabia as well. Ginger (*Zingiber officinale*) induces sweating, which helps cool the body during fever. It also contains many anti-inflammatory compounds, including some with mild aspirin-like effects. Thus, ginger may lower fever in more ways than one—it has both diaphoretic and anti-inflammatory effects. Several of these constituents in ginger have also shown to lower fever in animals.

☞ DIRECTIONS: Thinly slice a fresh ginger root (the root should be about the size of your thumb). Place the ginger in 1 quart of water. Bring to a boil, then simmer on the lowest possible heat for thirty minutes in a covered pot. Let cool for thirty more minutes. Strain and drink ½ to 1 cup, sweetened with honey. Repeat three times a day as desired. If you are pregnant, ask your doctor about taking ginger. As a precaution, don't take ginger in this dosage during pregnancy.

PEPPERMINT: Peppermint (*Mentha piperita*) is a folk remedy used for fever in Indiana and by some Hispanics in the Southwest. In China, cornmint (*Mentha arvensis*), a close relative of peppermint, is used in the same manner. Both plants, when taken as a hot tea, induce sweating, and help cool a fever. Cornmint and peppermint also contain large amounts of antiseptic and cooling menthol. In addition, as the steamy hot tea is drunk and the fragrance is inhaled, the menthol may act as a decongestant. Thus, this treatment might be best for treating fever accompanied by congestion.

☞ DIRECTIONS: Place ½ ounce of peppermint leaves in a 1-quart jar. Fill with boiling water and cover tightly. Let steep twenty minutes. While fever persists, strain and drink two or three cups a day. Wrap yourself in blankets and rest in bed after each cup.

ELDER FLOWERS AND BERRIES: Black elder *(Sambucus nigra)* is a famous flu and fever remedy from European traditional medicine. The plant's medicinal uses date back to the ancient Romans. Related elder species are native to North America. The Paiute and Shoshone Indians in the Rocky Mountains used the leaves and flowers of their local species for fevers, just as the Europeans used black elder. Elderberry was an official medicine in the *United States Pharmacopoeia* from the year of the book's founding in 1820 until 1909. The use of elder flower tea for fevers is still recorded in the folk medicine of the Amish, as well as in Indiana and by Hispanics in the Southwest.

The standard German medical textbook *Lehrbuch der Phytotherapie* describes elder as an immune stimulant. Elder flower tea is approved by the German government as a medicine for colds accompanied by cough. Recent research in Israel and Panama show that elderberry juice stimulates the immune system and can also significantly reduce the duration of an influenza attack.

The flowers contain anti-inflammatory constituents. (These constituents may also be present in other parts of the plant but have not yet been measured there. The bark and root of elder are very strong laxatives and should be

Starve a Fever

In the medicine of many North American Indian tribes, the standard treatment for fever was rest with either a liquid diet or no food at all. The admonition to "starve a fever" remains in many folk traditions today, including those of New England, the southern Appalachian mountains, and Indiana.

Starving a fever was also a firm tenet of early 20th century naturopathic medicine. Henry Lindlahr, M.D., N.D., the founder of a naturopathic medical school and a 200-patient nature cure hospital in Chicago, wrote in 1914 that a patient with a fever shouldn't eat "so much as a drop of milk" until the fever subsides. This approach, recorded in Lindlahr's book Natural Therapeutics (Volume II), has a sound physiological basis. Fasting reduces energy expenditures by the body that are normally required to produce digestive enzymes and absorb and eliminate the food. That energy can instead be used to fight the infection. Drinking plenty of liquids is important to prevent dehydration, however.

avoided.) The flowers are traditionally taken as a tea, while the berries are made into syrups. Taking too much elder tea, however, whether in the form of flowers or berries, can bring about a feeling of nausea.

☞ DIRECTIONS: Place ½ ounce of elder flowers in a 1-quart canning jar. Fill with boiling water. Cover and let steep for twenty minutes. Strain and pour a cup. Sweeten the tea with honey. Take a cup every four hours for a fever, especially one accompanying the flu. Wrap yourself in warm blankets after drinking the tea. If the tea gives you a queasy feeling after a few doses, take less or stop taking it completely.

CATNIP: A fever remedy from the Seventh Day Adventists calls for drinking catnip tea while soaking the feet in hot water. Catnip *(Nepeta cataria)* is also a fever remedy in the folk traditions of New England and Appalachia. Catnip's warming aromatic substances are diaphoretic and help induce a sweat. (Sticking the feet in hot water can induce sweating as well.) Catnip also purportedly acts as a sedative and may help you to rest and relax.

☞ DIRECTIONS: Fill the bathtub or a smaller tub with hot water. Put the feet in the water while drinking the hot tea. (This remedy is contraindicated in diabetics because of the possibility of burning the feet.)

To make the tea, pour boiling water over 1 ounce of catnip leaves in a 1-quart jar. Cover tightly and let steep for ten to fifteen minutes. As the fever persists, soak your feet every three to four hours while drinking half a cup of the tea.

FEVERFEW: European scientific research investigated the folk use of feverfew *(Tanacetum*

Herbs That'll Make You Sweat

Many traditional folk remedies for fever are called diaphoretics—plants or foods that make you sweat. Constituents in the plants increase the blood circulation to the skin, which causes you to sweat (sweating helps cool the body during a fever). It is essential to drink plenty of fluids when taking these herbs, however, or dehydration may result. Anise, boneset, catnip, cinnamon, elder, ginger, mint, thyme, and yarrow are all reported diaphoretics. Take them as hot teas, go to bed, and wrap yourself in warm blankets. Continue to drink plenty of fluids.

parthenium, Chrysan-
themum parthenium) in
the 1980s and early 1990s.
As a result, the herb be-
came popular in North
American health food
stores as a remedy for
migraine headache. Fever-
few is also famous in European and North American
folk medicine—particu-
larly in Indiana and Ap-
palachia—as a treatment
to lower fever (thus its
name), reduce arthritis
pain, or stimulate men-
struation.

Research shows that its
aromatic constituents
contain anti-inflammatory
properties that act simi-
larly to corticosteroid
drugs, although the con-
stituents are not nearly as
strong. The plant should
be used as fresh as pos-
sible. If dried leaves are
used, they should have a
strong aroma and be pre-
pared in a way that does
not evaporate the leaves'
aromatic constituents.

☞ DIRECTIONS: Place
½ ounce of feverfew leaves
in a 1-pint jar, fill with
boiling water, and cover
with a lid, tightly. Allow to
steep for thirty to forty
minutes. Drink half a cup
every three to four hours.

BONESET: Traditional
herbalist Tommie Bass
of northern Georgia, who
was the subject of a major
study of Appalachian folk
medicine during the 1980s,
named the herb boneset
(Eupatorium perfoliatum)
as his favorite fever
remedy. Boneset got its
English name in the 1700s
in Pennsylvania during an
influenza epidemic. The
flu was called "breakbone
fever" in that area; the
word breakbone referred to
the fever's accompanying
muscle aches and pains.
Boneset proved to "set the
bones" and relieve the
muscle discomfort. The
colonists learned the use
of the plant from the Cherokee and Iroquois Indians
and other eastern tribes.

Constituents have been
identified in boneset that
are both immune-stimu-
lating and anti-inflamma-
tory. Today, boneset is
used in the folk medicine
of Indiana and southern
continued on page 197

The Dead Lend a Hand

Although this may seem contradictory, folk medicine everywhere attributes special curative powers to corpses. Several reasons have been offered for this odd notion. In folk medicine, many remedies are opposites of their symptoms—such as when fullness is treated with bleeding or when irritating mustard plasters are applied to sore muscles. In the case of the corpse, it is believed that death may bring about health. It is also believed that the dead form a connection to the spiritual domain, and spirits are thought to be endowed with supernatural power.

The corpses that historically have received the most attention in folk medicine are those of executed criminals or suicides. This has led many scholars to suggest that, in folk medicine, untimely death is the major source of power. Many people believe humans have a pre-ordained life span. When death occurs prematurely, they imagine the vital, spiritual energy remains potent, at least until the time a person would have died naturally.

As is common throughout folk belief, powers that are effective in healing also have other uses—sometimes rather strange ones. The hand is the most common body part of the corpse used in healing. This use of the hand comes from a grisly and ancient idea called "the hand of glory." The hand of glory was a charm used by burglars, who believed it would make them invisible and prevent the occupants of a house from hearing any sounds they made. (In some versions, it was said that the charm would actually paralyze its victims.) The hand of glory was made by preserving the hand of a hanged criminal. Then a candle made from a corpse's fat would be placed in the hand and lit, or the fingers of the hand itself, soaked in fat, would be burned as candles! Most uses of the executed corpse were intended to heal rather than steal, however.

In Europe, the hangman was widely considered to have supernatural powers. This may have been because executions are a kind of sacrifice and, in a sense, the hangman represents God's authority in ending a life. Many hangmen advertised themselves as healers, and it was common for them to sell bits of clothing that belonged to the hanged criminal for magical and medical purposes. (Hangmen inherited the clothing as part of the payment for their grisly task.) Splinters from the gallows and the hangman's rope were also sold for healing purposes. Some hangmen would even permit parts of the hanged corpse to be taken.

In Pennsylvania and Ohio, the medicinal use of the hangman's rope was reported in both German and English tradition as a remedy for "fits" (seizures) and headache. The headache cure required that the noose be put around the patient's head! The use of gallow wood as a treatment for fever was recorded in Natural History, which was written in the first century A.D. by the Roman scholar and scientist Pliny the Elder. The use of gallow wood to treat fever continued in folk medicine.

In addition to the executions, suicides also have an important place in the folklore of premature death. In both Pennsylvania and Ohio the hanging rope of a suicide was believed to cure epilepsy.

Use of the dead in American folk medicine has its roots in European tradition. In this country, however, there were actually very few healing beliefs that involved a hanged corpse. This is probably because public hangings were practiced for a relatively brief time in America, and today only Delaware, Montana, New Hampshire, and Washington retain hanging as an official method of execution. Still, folklorists have found among Pennsylvania Germans the belief that a wen (a large sebaceous cyst) will go away if it is passed across the head of a recently hanged man.

In America, however, the most common "corpse medicine" involves ordinary dead bodies. Treatments often take place at wakes or viewings rather than executions. Remedies are usually for warts, goiters, wens, or tumors—things that need to be "taken away." Since the dead are "going away," these cures involve a sort of magical transference.

From the Midwest come two similar stories of such treatments. One account includes instructions for a cure: A fourteen-year-old girl went to where a corpse was laid out and rubbed her goiter three times with the corpse's hand, then returned the hand to its exact original position. Her goiter was said to be gone in a year. Another account explains that to rid yourself of a goiter you must use the hand from the same side of the corpse's body that your goiter is on. The remedy goes on to describe a person who used the left hand of a corpse to treat two goiters, one on each side. Only the goiter on the left side went away, confirming the tradition. This use of the dead hand for goiter seems very widespread and fairly current. Folk medicine scholar Wayland Hand tells of a woman with a noticeable goiter who was approached by a stranger who recommended that she treat the goiter by touching it with the hand of a corpse. This happened in California in the 1960s, and similar treatments have also been recorded in New York, Pennsylvania, Indiana, and Illinois.

Related beliefs for treating external tumors are widespread. However, sometimes the cure is a bit more complicated, as in this Pennsylvania German version: A string is tied around a dead man's finger. Then, the string is removed and tied around the tumor. As the string rots the tumor will disappear.

Other medicinal uses of the dead include placing a corpse's finger in the mouth for toothache (Alabama) and the general use of the dead man's hand to improve the complexion—by running the hand over moles, blackheads, and birthmarks.

Illinois as well as Appalachia. In Europe, boneset is used to treat colds and flu. Physicians in Germany use boneset to treat acute viral infections. Do not overdo it with boneset, however, because it can induce vomiting if taken in large quantities. Boneset was actually used for that purpose during the 18th and 19th centuries.

☞ DIRECTIONS: Place 1 teaspoon of dried boneset leaves in a cup and fill with boiling water. Let steep for fifteen minutes. Strain and drink the cup while still warm. Go to bed immediately and wrap yourself in warm blankets. Don't take more than one cup every four hours and no more than three cups a day. Stop taking boneset tea if you begin to feel nauseous.

LEMON BALM: In Indiana, lemon balm *(Melissa officinalis)* is a folk remedy for fever. The plant, which was native to southern Europe and northern Africa, arrived with the colonists and spread throughout North America. It has been used as a relaxing and sweat-inducing herb at least since the 12th century in Germany, where it is approved today as a medicine for digestive complaints or sleeping disorders, though not specifically for fevers. Of the sweat-inducing herbs included in this section, lemon balm is probably the mildest herb and is the most suitable for use in children. Lemon balm is also a mild sedative and can help relax the restless patient with cold or flu.

☞ DIRECTIONS: Pour boiling water over 1 teaspoon of the dried herb in a cup. Fill and let steep for ten minutes. While the tea is steeping, inhale the steam from the cup.

Strain and drink the tea, sweetened with honey as desired, up to four cups a day.

YARROW: The ancient Greeks used yarrow *(Achillea millefolium)* to reduce fevers. The plant's use has persisted in Europe ever since. At least 18 American Indian tribes from all corners of the continent also used yarrow (and its close botanical relatives) for the purpose of reducing fever. The early colonists throughout North America used yarrow to treat a wide variety of ailments—most of them infectious or inflammatory in nature. Using yarrow tea to fight colds and flu survives today in the folk medicine of New York, Appalachia, North Carolina, Indiana, and the American Southwest.

☞ DIRECTIONS: Place 1 ounce of dried or fresh yarrow in a 1-quart canning jar. Fill the jar with boiling water and cover tightly. Let steep for twenty minutes. Strain and pour a cup. Sweeten with honey.

Take two or three cups a day while fever persists. Wrap yourself in blankets and rest in bed after each cup.

WILLOW BARK: The Greeks used willow bark (*Salix spp.*) to treat pain more than 2,400 years ago. American Indians of the Alabama, Chickasaw, Houma, Montagnais, Shoshone, and Thompson tribes and the Ninivak Eskimos were using willow bark for the same purpose before the arrival of the European colonists. Scientific investigations of willow bark during the 19th century led to the isolation of its pain-relieving and fever-lowering constituents, and, ultimately, to the synthesis of aspirin in 1898. (Willow bark itself does not contain aspirin, but similar milder compounds.)

Willow bark is used to lower fever or reduce pain in the folk medicine of Indiana, New England, and the Southwest, as well as by professional medical herbalists of

North America and Great Britain. The German government has approved the use of willow bark by its conventional physicians for treating pain and fever. Besides its aspirin-like constituent salicin, willow bark contains other anti-inflammatory constituents as well.

☞ DIRECTIONS: Purchase some willow bark capsules in a health food store or herb shop. Take as directed on the label. Alternately, place 2 teaspoons of powdered willow bark in a cup, fill with boiling water, and let steep for fifteen to twenty minutes. Sweeten with honey as desired, and drink up to four cups a day for as long as the fever persists.

DANDELION: A common herb used to reduce fever in Chinese folk medicine is dandelion. (In traditional Chinese medicine, dandelion is classified as a "heat clearing" herb.) The Chinese dandelion (*Taraxacum mongolici*) and this country's common backyard dandelion (*Tarax-*

acum officinale) have similar appearances and constituents. Like many of the herbs in this category, dandelion contains several anti-inflammatory constituents. But, unlike the other herbs listed above, dandelion does not induce sweating. Its fever-reducing activity, if any, comes from some other mechanism. Dandelion has not been tested for fever-lowering properties by conventional scientists.

☞ DIRECTIONS: Pick some dandelions, taking the whole root and leaf. (Be sure to harvest them away from lawns or fields that may have been sprayed with chemical pesticides.) Wash the roots well with running water. Place 1 to 2 ounces of the plant in 1 quart of water. Bring to a boil and cover. Simmer on the lowest heat for thirty to forty minutes. When suffering from fever, drink the quart in 3 to 4 doses during the course of a day. If your fever is not better within three days, be sure to see a doctor. Don't take dandelion if you suffer from indigestion or heartburn.

AMERICAN GINSENG: Another herb used to treat feverish illnesses in Chinese folk medicine is American ginseng *(Panax quinquefolium)*. It is also used by residents of Appalachia.

Although American ginseng has never been used much in American medicine, it is a very popular remedy in China. Hundreds of tons of American ginseng are shipped from farms in Michigan and Wisconsin to China every year. (American ginseng, also reputed for its sedating effects, is often more popular than Asian ginseng in Chinatowns throughout North America.) The Chinese use the American ginseng species for different purposes than their own native Asian ginseng *(Panax ginseng)*. They view American ginseng as a "cooling" plant; they take it during hot summer weather and to cool feverish illnesses. Other than the basic identification of its constituents, very little scientific research has investigated American ginseng. Its "cooling" properties have not been examined or demonstrated.

☞ DIRECTIONS: Chop 3½ ounces of ginseng and place in 1 quart of liquor such as vodka. Cover and let stand for five or six weeks in a cool dark place, turning the jar frequently. When fighting a fever, take 1 ounce after dinner or before bed.

LEMON: Lemons in the form of hot lemonade is a folk remedy for fever and influenza in New England and Indiana. The ancient Romans used lemons in the same way. No one has performed clinical trials to see if this method really works, but the constituents of lemon and its fragrant oils may indeed be helpful for treating fever and infection.

Lemon juice is an expectorant, increasing the flow of healthy mucus to infected mucous membranes.

Mal Ojo

In the Hispanic traditions of the American Southwest, the "mal ojo" or "evil eye" is believed to be one possible cause of high fever. "Ojo" can occur when a person with a powerful gaze looks admiringly at someone without touching them. Children are most susceptible.

The symptoms of ojo can include sudden onset of high fever, vomiting, headache, fainting, or convulsions. The diagnosis of ojo can be made by examining the contents of a fresh egg that's broken after it's passed over the patient's body. If the contents of the egg appear to be cooked, or the yolk appears to have the image of an eye, the person is a victim of the strong person's gaze. The perpetrator must touch the patient as soon as possible to cure the condition. Various methods are used if that individual is not available. The condition caused by mal ojo can be prevented by making sure that, if a child is complimented, the caregiver is sure to touch him or her.

Other constituents of lemon are antimicrobial and anti-inflammatory. It is not known whether clinically significant levels of these constituents are present in hot lemonade, however.

☞ DIRECTIONS: Pour 1 cup of boiling water over a blended whole lemon—skin, pulp, and all. Let the mixture steep for five minutes. While the tea is steeping, inhale the fumes. Drink one cup. Do this at first onset of a fever, and repeat three to four times a day for the duration of the infection.

ONIONS: Although onions (*Allium cepa*) appear to be a near-universal remedy for treating fever, recommendations for their use vary. In folk medicine, it has been recommended that onion slices be placed on the bottoms of the feet;

put under the bed; eaten raw, roasted, or boiled; taken in teas, milk, or wine; worn in the sock or in a bag around the neck; or applied to the chest as a poultice. In every region of the country, American Indians used wild onions to lower fever. The use of onions continues today in the folk traditions of New England, New York, North Carolina, Appalachia, Indiana, and China.

The onion's constituents may explain its widespread use for treating fever, colds, and flu. Onions are also expectorant—they induce the flow of healthy and cleansing mucus. It is possible that, in the traditional "chicken soup" cure for the common cold, it is the onion that actually does the trick, not the chicken!

☞ DIRECTIONS: Cut up 1 whole large onion, and simmer in a covered pot for twenty minutes. Drink a cup of the tea three to four times a day while your fever lasts. After each cup, go to bed, wrap yourself in blankets, and keep warm.

REACTIVE HYDRO-THERAPY: Here is a fever-reducing method from Gypsy traditions that is taught in North American naturopathic medical colleges. This type of treatment—which includes warm coverings over mild cold applications—is called *reactive hydrotherapy*. In reactive hydrotherapy, the body reacts to a mild cold application by sending blood to the area of the cold stimulus.

☞ DIRECTIONS: Take cotton socks, soak them in cold water, wring them out, and put them on the patient's feet. Cover the cold socks with one or two pair of warm wool socks. Leave in place for at least forty minutes, or overnight.

BLANKETS: A tradition from North Carolina calls for simply wrapping the patient in warm blankets and putting him to bed. When you wrap the patient warmly, his body does not have to work as hard to produce a fever. (Normally the body has to produce shivers and chills to raise the temperature. The blankets reduce the need for this.) Plus, rest in bed conserves energy and frees the body to fight infection.

☞ DIRECTIONS: Comfortably wrap the patient in 1 to 3 layers of blankets, and let him quietly rest in bed.

❧ Foot Problems ❧

◼ ◼ ◼

The most common foot problem mentioned in the literature of folk medicine is athlete's foot, a fungal infection of the feet. The organisms that cause athlete's foot normally reside on the skin but thrive in a hot, moist setting. An actual outbreak of athlete's foot may be due to either poor hygiene—failing to keep the feet clean and dry—or to a systemic weakness of the immune system.

Antifungal creams and ointments as well as improved foot hygiene make up the conventional treatment for athlete's foot. Many of the folk remedies for athlete's foot increase local circulation to the feet, thus increasing the presence of the body's own blood-borne immune agents that help fight infection. Other folk treatments include antifungal and anti-infective herbs and foods. These folk remedies are effective against the most common infecting organisms— members of the *Trichophyton* and *Microsporum* genera of fungi—but are ineffective against many other infectious agents. Some of the folk remedies to follow may be more effective than others. For example, the garlic foot bath may be more effective than some of the recommended creams and ointments, because garlic kills a wider range of organisms. Garlic and other antiseptic herbs may also kill the bacteria that can infect and complicate a case of athlete's foot.

Other foot problems covered in this section include cold feet and in-grown toenails. Proper methods to rewarm cold feet were of great interest to our ancestors because many of them worked as farmers, often in cold temperatures. You'll also discover a few treatments for curing ingrown toenails. (If a stubborn ingrown toenail causes persistent discomfort, however, a visit to a podiatrist—a foot doctor—may be in order.)

Remedies

ATHLETE'S FOOT

PLANTAIN: A favorite remedy for foot infections among American Indians of the Southwest is plan-tain *(Plantago major)*. (Plantain is used in many cultures to treat wounds, bites, and stings.) Plantain leaf contains several iden-

Keep Your Feet Dry

Both conventional and folk medicine alike recommend keeping the feet dry to prevent the development of ath-lete's foot. Here's a prevention program from New England folk medicine for doing just that: Wash the feet thoroughly, dry them, and change socks twice a day. Each time you wash your feet, dust them with cornstarch, which will absorb moisture. If the feet still get wet or sweaty, dry them more often. Also, rotate wearing two pairs of shoes, allowing each pair to dry for a full twenty-four hours before wearing them again. You can also keep shoes dry by dusting the insides with cornstarch.

tified anti-inflammatory and bacterial properties as well as analgesic and antiseptic properties. It also contains the constituent allantoin, which promotes cell proliferation and tissue healing. This four-leaved plant is a common weed found in lawns and along sidewalks throughout North America.

☞ DIRECTIONS: Crush fresh plantain leaves and rub the juice directly onto the infected area.

ALOE VERA: Although aloe vera juice is best known for its ability to treat burns, it is also recognized as a folk cure for athlete's foot. In experiments testing aloe vera's ability to heal burns, scientists found that the plant juice not only promoted the growth of healthy tissue, but also acted as a disinfectant, reducing bacterial counts in the burns. Both of these properties are also beneficial for treating athlete's foot.

☞ DIRECTIONS: Break off a part of the leaf. Apply the juicy sap to the infected area. If you don't grow your own aloe vera plant, you can purchase aloe vera gel at a health food store or drugstore.

GARLIC: Calvin Thrash, M.D., and Agatha Thrash, M.D., teachers of the folk remedies of the Seventh Day Adventist religion, suggest that garlic water can cure a fungal infection. Scientific experiments have shown that garlic's main antimicrobial constituent, allicin, kills more than 40 different types of bacteria, viruses, molds, fungi, and parasites. In fact, allicin is the plant's natural defense against the microorganisms that attack it! Allicin seems to work against most of the organisms that attack humans as well. The allicin is only released when a clove is cut, crushed, or otherwise broken apart. Thus, the best method for releasing the maximum amount of allicin is to pulverize the garlic cloves in a blender. A hot garlic-water foot-bath helps soften the superficial layers of the skin so the garlic can penetrate to the full depth of the infection. The hot water and the mild irritation of the garlic also draw circulation to the feet, enhancing local immune resistance in the area.

☞ DIRECTIONS: Blend 2 whole garlic bulbs in a blender and add to 1 quart of hot water. (The bulbs do not have to be peeled.) Fill a small tub with enough hot water so that the feet will be covered. Add the quart of hot garlic water to the bath. Soak the feet for twenty minutes, once a day, in the evening. Towel the feet briskly after the treatment to brush away any dead skin and dry the feet.

LICKING YOUR WOUNDS: A folk remedy from contemporary Indiana suggests the cure for athlete's foot is letting a dog lick your feet. As outrageous as this may seem, allowing dogs to disinfect your wounds with their saliva is a widespread practice throughout the world and has been practiced among North American Indian tribes and by Europeans at least since the 1500s. Modern science also supports the use of dog saliva.

Saliva is part of the immune system, and it contains a number of antimicrobial substances, including those with such names as mucin, fibronectin, beta-2 microglobulin, lactoferrin, salivary peroxidase, histatin, and cystatin. (These antimicrobial substances are part of the reason why dogs can eat substances right off the street or out of a neighbor's garbage can and not get sick.) Another antibacterial substance found in saliva, lysozyme, has been developed into a drug for commercial use in Europe for treating wounds and infections. Saliva also contains antibodies. Finally, saliva contains healing agents that promote the growth of new cells. These saliva-based growth factors are being tested by pharmaceutical companies for possible use as wound-healing drugs.

☞ DIRECTIONS: Take off your shoes and socks, wash your feet, and let your dog start licking.

BLEACH: A remedy for athlete's foot from New England is to soak the feet in bleach water once a day. The same remedy was recommended by the naturopathic physician John Bastyr in the 1980s. Bastyr Health Sciences University in Seattle was named after this doctor, whose medical career—which included the use of natural remedies—spanned more than sixty years.

☞ DIRECTIONS: Using ¼ cup of bleach for each quart of water, prepare enough bleach water to cover the feet in a small tub. Soak for fifteen to twenty minutes.

URINE: Fungal infections of various sorts are sometimes treated in the folk medicine of New England, the Southwest, and the Midwest with urine. Urine therapy for cleansing wounds and treating a variety of infections has appeared in the ancient medical systems of Mexico, Egypt, Persia, India, and China. The remedy was even used in Europe in the 17th and 18th centuries. During World War II in North Africa, British soldiers were shocked to see their Arab allies urinating on the wounds of injured soldiers.

Modern science suggests reasons why urine may be an effective disinfectant. Urine from a healthy person is as sterile as boiled water; therefore, it is safe to put on an infected area of the skin. Urine also contains the substance urea, a disinfectant used today in pharmaceutical preparations to clean and disinfect burns and wounds. Urea has strong drying properties and kills fungi, bacteria, and viruses by literally sucking the water right out of them. (If you are revolted by the idea of putting urine on the skin, consider this: Many modern cosmetic skincare products contain urea derived from the urine of cows.)

☞ DIRECTIONS: Cover the infected areas of your feet with your own urine each time you urinate. A recommendation from New England says not to wash off the urine for several days in a row.

COLD FEET

HOT FOOT BATH: Perhaps the most obvious treatment for cold feet, once back indoors, is to soak them in warm water. A hydrotherapy treatment from German immigrants at the turn of the century called for a 15 minute bath

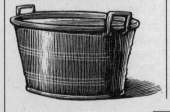

in 102°F water. It's best to measure the temperature of the water with a thermometer, however. Don't just stick your feet right in because the temperature-sensing nerves of cold feet may not be able to detect if the water is too hot.

☞ DIRECTIONS: Run hot bath water in a small tub or bathtub. Measure the temperature of the water with a thermometer, and then add cold water until the temperature is about 102°F degrees. Soak the feet for fifteen minutes.

RED PEPPERS: A suggestion from North Carolina folklore for warming cold feet for those who must remain outdoors for work or play is to put red pepper pods in the shoes. The mild irritation of the capsaicin in peppers draws warming blood to the area. Capsaicin also alleviates local pain. Recent studies show that capsaicin can deplete substance P, which is involved in pain transmission. Hispanic cowboys from the Southwest often use powdered cayenne pepper *(Capsicum annuum)* instead of the unbroken pods.

☞ DIRECTIONS: Sprinkle a small amount of cayenne pepper in your socks before going out into the cold. Bring a clean pair of socks along just in case the red pepper becomes irritating or painful. Commercial capsaicin ointment is also available for topical application to control pain from shingles and arthritis.

CINNAMON: Much of China endures cold winters, so Chinese folk traditions have a lot to say about cold feet. Most Chinese preventives and remedies for cold feet are herbs that stimulate circulation. The Chinese recommend cinnamon *(Cinnamomum cassia),* taken internally, to prevent cold hands and feet in those who work outdoors or who have cold dispositions.

☞ DIRECTIONS: Stir 1 gram of powdered cinnamon (the amount in two average-size gelatin capsules) into a glass of hot water and let steep for a few minutes. Drink three times a day.

GINSENG: A famous remedy from China for rewarming cold limbs is Asian ginseng *(Panax ginseng).* In traditional Chinese medicine, ginseng is indicated for those men or women who are run down and fatigued and who also feel cold and have cold hands and feet. Animal experiments have demonstrated that Asian ginseng helps the body to resist chilling and hypothermia.

☞ DIRECTIONS: During the winter months, purchase an Asian ginseng product at a health food store, herb shop, or Chinese or Korean market. The potency of commercial ginseng products varies widely, but the rule of thumb is that you will have to buy a more expensive product if you want to get good results. (Cheap ginseng products tend to contain almost no ginseng.) On the other hand, beware of paying for expensive "rare" ginseng roots, a scam common in some herb shops. And make sure that you are buying Asian ginseng, and not American ginseng *(Panax quinque-folius)* or Siberian ginseng *(Eleutherococcus senti-cosus* or *Acanthopanax senticosus),* which have different medicinal properties. A top-of-the-line encapsulated product is probably your best buy. Take 1 to 3 grams a day during the winter months.

INGROWN TOENAILS

HOT SOAK AND A TRIM: Here's a treatment for ingrown toenails from folklorist Clarence Meyer's *American Folk Medicine.*
☞ DIRECTIONS: Soak the foot in hot soapy water for fifteen minutes, until the nail becomes soft. With a knife, scrape the nail until it is very thin on the upper surface. This will supposedly cause the nail to assume its proper shape and flatten out.

YARN: An ingrown toenail treatment from New England calls for raising the toenail up from the nail bed with a piece of yarn.
☞ DIRECTIONS: Using a piece of wool yarn like dental floss, work it as deeply as possible under the corner of the toenail that's growing inward. Cut the yarn and leave it in place. This will make that corner of the nail grow straight. If in doubt, or to avoid infection, however, you may want to consult a podiatrist.

❧ Headaches ❧

■ ■ ■

A headache is a symptom of disease, and not a disease in itself. Rarely is a headache the symptom of a serious illness—most headaches are caused by minor conditions, such as muscle tension in the neck and around the skull or inflammation of blood vessels in the brain.

There are three basic types of headaches. The vascular headache occurs when blood vessels in the head enlarge and press on nerves, causing pain. The most common vascular headache is the migraine. The second type of headache is the muscle contraction headache, which results when the muscles of the face, neck, or scalp contract and tighten. A tension headache is an example of a muscle contraction headache. The third kind of headache is the inflam-matory headache. Such a headache is the result of pressure within the head. The causes range from relatively minor conditions, such as sinusitis, to more serious problems, such as brain tumors.

Headaches are most often treated with aspirin and nonsteroidal anti-inflammatory drugs (NSAIDs) such as ibuprofen. Treatment of a migraine already in progress usually consists of a drug therapy program chosen from a variety of painkillers, sedatives, and special drugs and remedies, including vasoconstricting drugs and caffeine. Tension headaches can be treated by eliminating the tension or correcting the physical problem that is causing the headaches. This can some-times be done through physical manipulation of the spine or skull by a chiropractic or osteopathic physician.

The herbal folk remedies for headaches, which are still used today by alternative physicians in the United States and by some conventional doctors in Europe, fall into four categories: pain-relievers, anti-inflammatories, sedatives, and digestive herbs. The pain-relieving and anti-inflammatory herbs may relieve most types of headaches. The sedatives work well for relieving tension headaches. The digestive herbs and laxatives are most useful for treating headaches that accompany digestive problems.

Remedies

WILLOW BARK: More than 2,400 years ago, the Greeks used willow bark (*Salix spp.*) to treat headache pain. American Indians of the Alabama, Chickasaw, Houma, Montagnais, Shoshone, and Thompson tribes and the Ninivak Eskimos used it for the same purpose, even before the arrival of the European colonists. Willow bark is still used to treat

Feverfew?

Scientific studies in the 1980s popularized the use of the herb feverfew (*Tanacetum parthenium*) for treating migraines. But think twice before investing large amounts of money in this herb, however. Although it proved more effective than the placebo in the clinical trials, feverfew actually helped fewer than half of the people who took it—and it didn't even help them very much. In fact, for most people, it didn't prevent migraines at all. It only reduced their occurrence—from four migraines a month to three. Besides, further studies have demonstrated that the active constituent in feverfew (the one that helps lessen migraine occurrences) is not even present in most commercial products.

headache pain in the folk medicine of Indiana, New England, and the Southwest. It is recommended by professional medical herbalists of North America and Great Britain. The German government has approved its use by conventional physicians for treating pain and fever.

The most important active constituent in willow bark is salicin, but the bark also contains at least three other anti-inflammatory constituents. In Germany, the suggested

Where Aspirin Came From

Aspirin is perhaps the best-known drug for treating headaches in North America today. In fact, per-capita consumption of aspirin in the United States is one tablet per person per week. Aspirin was "discovered" after chemists studied plants such as willow bark, sage, and pennyroyal. These plants, and others, have traditionally been used to treat pain.

The first of the plants to be studied was willow bark, which had been used by both the ancient Greeks and by the American Indians to treat pain. The pain-relieving constituent of willow bark, salicin, was isolated in the 19th century. Similar aspirin-like compounds were later found in other plants as well. In fact, chemists created acetylsalicylic acid—aspirin—from salicylic acid obtained from meadowsweet.

Further study in the 20th century has led to a whole new class of drugs, called nonsteroidal anti-inflammatory drugs (NSAIDs), which have anti-inflammatory properties similar to those of aspirin. NSAIDs are useful in the treatment of athletic injuries, postoperative pain, rheumatoid and osteoarthritis, and skin, bone, and teeth disorders. We owe our knowledge of this new class of medicines to the original folk use of plants for pain.

dose is about one gram of the powdered bark—the amount in about two average-sized gelatin capsules. Willow bark is not as potent as aspirin, but it is less likely to cause stomach upset.

☞ DIRECTIONS: To make a tea, place 2 teaspoons of powdered willow bark in a cup and fill with boiling water. Let steep for fifteen to twenty minutes. Sweeten with honey as desired. Drink up to 4 cups a day. Note that salicin can cause skin rashes in some people.

Alternately, you can purchase willow bark capsules in a health food store or an herb shop. Take as directed on the product label.

ROSEMARY AND SAGE: A folk remedy for treating headache pain is to drink a tea of rosemary *(Rosmarinus officinalis)* and sage *(Salvia officinalis)*. Rosemary has been a popular medicine in Europe for treating pain at least since the time of the ancient Greeks. Among

the Greeks, rosemary had a reputation for improving the memory.

Today, rosemary is used to soothe headaches in the folk medicine of China, and, in the United States, it is used for the same purpose in Indiana and among the Amish. The German government has approved the use of rosemary for pain. There, rosemary is often used externally, in preparations such as salves and baths. It is a common folk use to apply rosemary to the temples in the form of a poultice to relieve headache pain. Sage is not often used in folk medicine as a pain reliever, but it has an important chemical constituent in common with rosemary—rosmarinic acid (see sidebar, "Rosmarinic Acid," page 215). In addition, the combination of rosemary and sage contains more than 20 anti-inflammatory constituents, although some of these exist only in minute amounts. Seek medical attention for any headache that lasts longer than three days. Do not ingest rosemary in any amount exceeding those usually found in foods because of the herb's reputed abortifacient and emmenagogue effects.

☞ DIRECTIONS: Place 1 teaspoon of crushed rosemary leaves and 1 teaspoon of crushed sage leaves in a cup. Fill with boiling water. Cover well to prevent the escape of volatile substances. Let steep until the tea reaches room temperature. Take ½-cup doses two or three times a day for two or three days. You don't have to mix rosemary and sage to find pain relief. You can also try drinking either rosemary or sage teas separately.

AMERICAN PENNYROYAL: Pennyroyal tea (Hedeoma pulegioides) is a headache remedy of the Onondaga Indians. In European folk medicine, a European species of pennyroyal (Mentha pulegioides L.) is used for pain relief. In fact, the 17th century British herbalist John Gerard wrote of pennyroyal: "A Garland of Pennie Royall made and worne about the

Rosmarinic Acid

Rosmarinic acid is a nonsteroidal anti-inflammatory agent similar to aspirin, ibuprofen, and acetaminophen. High amounts of rosmarinic acid are contained in many plants used in folk medicine to treat pain, including rosemary, sage, mint, basil, and thyme. Some folk traditions advise crushing these plants (to release the rosmarinic acid) and applying the plant material to the temples or forehead. This type of application may sound somewhat odd, but animal studies have shown that rosmarinic acid is readily absorbed through the skin. You can add rosemary to your bathwater as well. The German government has approved the use of rosemary as a topical agent for pain relief.

Using Your Head

A German herbal that was used by turn-of-the-century immigrants suggested binding mint across the forehead, a practice that American Indians also used for treating headache pain. Folk traditions from every region of North America and Europe recommend applying substances to the head to treat headaches. For example, from New England to the Southwest, folk remedies suggest applying camphor spirits and vinegar to the head to treat headache pain. In New England, practitioners of folk medicine apply witch hazel to the forehead or spread sauerkraut on the temples. Other North American traditions call for applying raw onions or boneset leaves to the forehead. We don't know if any of these methods really works, but some medicinal substances, such as the anti-inflammatory rosmarinic acid found in mint, are easily absorbed through the skin.

head is of great force against swimming in the head, and the paines and giddiness thereof." The use of pennyroyal for treating headaches persists today in the folk medicine of Appalachia and Indiana. Pennyroyal contains significant amounts of the anti-inflammatory substance diosmin.

☞ DIRECTIONS: Place 1 teaspoon of dried pennyroyal leaves in a cup and fill with boiling water.

Cover well to avoid the loss of volatile constituents. Let steep. Take ½-cup doses, up to four times a day. Seek medical attention for any headache that lasts longer than three days.

MINTS: The mints—peppermint (Mentha piperita) and spearmint (Mentha spicata)—are used as headache remedies in the folk medicine of the particular regions where continued on page 218

The Evil Eye

◈ ◈ ◈

One of the most widespread folk beliefs in the world is the belief in the power of the "evil eye." Although explanations vary slightly, most people who hold this belief say that certain individuals have the power to cause evil to others just by way of looking at them. The person who casts the evil eye may not even know they are doing it. The most common cause for "overlooking," or putting a spell on someone, is envy. For example, if someone with "the power" envies another's good fortune, she may put the gaze on the person she envies. Her power results in bad luck or ill health for the person she "overlooked."

Children and pregnant women are considered to be likely targets for this kind of cursing. Praising a child without also touching or pinching him can be seen as a dangerous action. Sometimes a person who has complimented a child will spit to stop any unintentional envy she may be feeling.

The evil eye is a supernatural method of causing illness. As a result, virtually all preventions and treatments for evil eye also involve supernatural beliefs and practices. Cures are usually performed by women who have had the healing secrets told to them by older healers.

A wide variety of charms can be used to deflect the power of the evil eye. An amulet in the shape of an eye or a red horn can be worn as a defense. Garlic, salt, or written copies of religious texts can also be worn.

Hand gestures are among the most common ways of warding off "wasting sickness" or bad luck associated with the evil eye. Here's one gesture you can use: Point down with your index finger and pinkie finger extended straight and your thumb holding the middle two fingers down.

Water Treatments

A variety of "water cures" for headaches are mentioned in North American folk literature. Little consistency exists between the treatments, however. For instance, Indiana folklore suggests applying a hot cloth to the forehead. New England tradition suggests applying cold water or ice to the area. Perhaps the method that makes the most sense for migraines—a method that is recommended by the Amish and is also taught in today's North American naturopathic medical colleges—is the hot foot bath. When heat is applied to the feet, it increases blood circulation there, moving blood away from the dilated vessels in the brain and easing the head pain. Sometimes a cold cloth is applied to the head, or a few teaspoons of mustard powder are added to the foot bath, to reinforce the action.

they grow. American Indians of both eastern and western North America, including the Cherokee, Iroquois, Gosuite, and Paiute tribes, used these mints as headache remedies. Some tribes crushed the plant and inhaled the fumes; others placed the plant on the forehead in the same way rosemary is used (see "Rosemary and Sage," page 214).

Today, mints are used in the folk medicine of China, Mexico, Appalachia, and the American Southwest to treat headaches. The mints contain about the same levels of the anti-inflammatory rosmarinic acid as do rosemary and sage (see sidebar, "Rosmarinic Acid," page 215).

☞ DIRECTIONS: Place 1 ounce of dried mint leaves in a 1-quart jar and fill with boiling water. Cover tightly to prevent the escape of the aromatic constituents. The dose is ½ cup of tea, two to four times a day. If a headache persists for more than three days, a visit to the doctor is in order.

COFFEE AND TEA: Coffee and tea are recommended as headache cures in several traditions. Caffeine is the medicinal constituent responsible for the benefits. Caffeine is also used in conventional medicine to treat migraine headaches. It works by constricting the vessels of the brain, which are sometimes dilated during a headache attack. Tea is recommended in New England, and strong black coffee in Appalachia. Black coffee is a famous cure throughout Europe and North America for the type of headache that accompanies hangover. Note that habitual use of caffeine can cause headache on withdrawal, however.

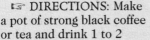

☞ DIRECTIONS: Make a pot of strong black coffee or tea and drink 1 to 2 cups to relieve an acute headache.

YARROW: Yarrow (*Achillea millefolium*) has been used as a universal pain and headache remedy among various American Indian tribes, including the Cheyenne, Chippewa, Gosuite, Iroquois, Lummi, Mendocino, Navaho, Paiute, Seneca, and Shoshone. Yarrow contains at least 18 anti-inflammatory constituents, including salicylic acid, an aspirin-like substance.

☞ DIRECTIONS: Place 1 ounce of dried or fresh yarrow leaves in a 1-quart jar and fill with boiling water. Cover tightly to prevent the escape of the aromatic constituents. The dose is one-half cup of the tea, two to four times a day. If any headache persists for more than three days, see your doctor.

LAXATIVES: A collection of remedies by folklorist Clarence Meyer called

American Folk Medicine suggests taking low doses of laxatives to cure a headache. This remedy is best used on headaches that accompany constipation. The habitual use of laxatives is not recommended, however.

☞ DIRECTIONS: Place ¼ teaspoon of senna leaves in a cup. Add ¼ teaspoon of sage leaves and ¼ teaspoon of powdered ginger. Fill the cup with boiling water. Let steep until cool. Drink a cup every four hours. Do not exceed 3 doses in a day. Do not repeat the treatment for a second day. If the constipation and headache persist, see a physician. Do not use laxatives during pregnancy.

BONESET: During the 1700s, the herb boneset *(Eupatorium perfoliatum)* was one of the most common household remedies in the eastern colonies. The colonists learned the plant's uses from the American Indians, who used it to treat a wide variety of conditions, including colds, flu, and arthritis pain. The use of boneset for headaches, especially migraine headaches, persists today in southern Appalachia and in Indiana.

Several constituents of boneset have been shown to be anti-inflammatory, but their clinical significance is not clear. Boneset contains bitter substances that promote the secretion of digestive enzymes, so boneset can be used as a mild laxative. Thus, boneset may be most appropriate for headaches that accompany or follow digestive disturbances.

☞ DIRECTIONS: Place 1 tablespoon of dried boneset leaves in a cup and fill with boiling water. Let stand until cool (room temperature). Strain and drink the liquid in 3 divided doses during the day, away from meals. Note: Boneset taken in larger doses has been shown to cause nausea.

WORMWOOD: Plants of the *Artemisia* genus *(Artemisia spp.)* have been used as pain remedies by at

Vinegar and Brown Paper

Using vinegar to treat headaches is a common remedy in traditional folk culture throughout the eastern United States. North Carolina folklore suggests wetting a brown paper bag with vinegar and placing it on the head. Some North Carolina variations of the remedy call for using a vinegar-soaked towel instead of a paper bag, but the paper bag method also appears in Amish folklore and in the remedies of contemporary Indiana folk medicine. A Vermont method is to drink the vinegar—a tablespoon in a glass of water along with a tablespoon of honey. Another Indiana method is to mix equal parts of water and vinegar, bring to a boil, and inhale the vapor, taking 75 breaths. There is no apparent scientific rationale for any of these practices.

least 22 American Indian tribes throughout North America. Some tribes received the pain-relieving properties of the plants by burning them and inhaling their smoke and aromatic oils. To treat a headache, others made a tea of the leaves and used them as a wash on the forehead and temples. The use of the *Artemisia* species is recorded today in the folk medicine of northern New Mexico. The European species *Artemisia absinthum* (or wormwood) is approved as a digestive stimulant by the German government. Excessive use in large amounts can lead to brain damage, however.

The active constituents of plants in the Artemisia species include bitter digestive stimulants and anti-inflammatory volatile oils such as azulenes. These constituents are also present in yarrow and chamomile.

☞ DIRECTIONS: Place 1 teaspoon of wormwood

Bitter Herbs for Healing

Many traditional folk remedies for headaches require the use of bitter herbs. Such traditional medical systems as Ayurveda (from India), Unani Tibb (from Arabia), and traditional Chinese medicine consider the bitter flavor of the herbs to be "cooling." In these systems of medicine, inflammatory headaches such as migraines are universally treated with bitter digestive herbs. The concept is that the herbs cool the "fire" in the digestive system and prevent it from "rising" to the head and causing a headache. Bitter herbs in this section include yarrow, senna, boneset, hop, and chamomile.

leaves in a cup of water and fill with boiling water. Cover well. Let cool to room temperature. Take ½-cup doses every three hours for up to three days. If the headache persists, see a doctor.

HOP: The herb hop (*Humulus lupulus*), which is responsible for the bitter flavor of beer, has been used as a pain reliever by the Cherokee, Dakota, and Mohegan Indian tribes. It is approved by the German government for use as a sedative and may be best suited to relieving stress-related headaches or headaches that interfere with sleep.

☞ DIRECTIONS: Place 1 teaspoon of hop flowers in a cup and add boiling water. Cover and let stand for ten minutes. Drink two or three cups a day for up to three days.

Also, you can crush 1 ounce of dried hop flowers, sprinkle with alcohol, and place inside a pillow. Sleep with the pillow close to the face.

CHAMOMILE: Chamomile tea (*Matricaria recutita*) is recommended for headaches today in the Hispanic folk medicine of the Southwest. Chamomile contains bitter digestive stimulants, anti-inflammatory compounds, and sedative constituents. It may be especially appropriate for soothing stress-related headaches. Other activities of chamomile tea have shown to have antibacterial, anti-inflammatory, antispasmodic, and antiviral properties.

☞ DIRECTIONS: Place ½ ounce of the flowers in a 1-quart jar. Fill the jar with boiling water and cover. Let steep until the tea reaches room temperature. To soothe a headache, strain and drink ½-cup doses every three hours.

❧ Hemorrhoids ❧

■ ■ ■

In some cases, hemorrhoids are the result of poor toilet habits. Habitual postponement of bowel movements can lead to loss of rectal function and undesirable straining during elimination. Straining puts increased pressure on the veins and slows the flow of blood, thereby contributing to swelling and inflammation of the veins. If bowel movements are postponed, the stools retained in the bowels may lose moisture. When feces becomes dry and hard, the added strain of constipation favors the development of hemorrhoids.

Another source of hemorrhoidal irritation comes from pressure on the veins due to disease of the liver or heart or due to a tumor. Pregnancy may also contribute to the development of hemorrhoids, because the enlarged uterus increases pressure on the veins. Diet also plays a major role in the development of hemorrhoids. A diet containing a high proportion of refined foods, rather than foods with natural roughage, increases the likelihood of constipation, and therefore, the likelihood of hemorrhoids. And lack of exercise is one of the strongest contributing factors to the formation of hemorrhoids because exercise ensures robust circulation in the abdominal venous system.

Hemorrhoids occur "universally," according to *The Merck Manual,* a standard medical text. If they do not cause pain or other symptoms, no treatment or surgical removal is necessary. Conventional treatments include giving bulk laxatives to soften the stool (see "Constipation," page 121), warm sitz baths, topical anesthetics for itching or pain, and witch hazel compresses (a remedy we adopted from the American Indians). Other treatments include tying off the hemorrhoids and removing the hemor-

rhoids by surgical means. Folk remedies include all of these treatments—except the tying off procedure and the surgery. In folk medicine, the laxative effect is often achieved by taking certain herbs or foods.

Remedies

WITCH HAZEL EXTRACT: A commercial witch hazel extract *(Hamamelis virginiana)* has been a popular over-the-counter remedy for hemorrhoids in North America since the mid-1800s. The story of this commercial product is one of the best documented cases of an American Indian medicine that was adopted by both the medical profession and the general public. In the early 1840s, Theron Pond of Utica, New York, saw the local Indians of the Oneida tribe using an herbal preparation to treat burns, boils, wounds, and other afflictions of the skin. After making the acquaintance of their medicine man, Pond learned that the preparation was made by steeping witch hazel bark in an ordinary tea kettle over an open fire and collecting the steam. The result was a clear liquid with a golden color and strong aroma. Pond went into partnership with the medicine man to produce the product for local sales. They added alcohol to stabilize the product. Called Golden Treasure, the product was put on the market in 1848. Pond died a few years later and, ultimately, the product was renamed Pond's Extract.

Salves

Salves, often called ointments, are fat-based preparations used to soothe abrasions, heal wounds and lacerations, protect babies' skin from diaper rash, and soften dry, rough skin and chapped lips. Homemade salves are also widespread among the folk treatments for hemorrhoids. Salves are made by heating an herb with fat or vegetable oil until the fat absorbs the plant's healing properties. These salves can be quite easily made from lard or butter, which are the most common ingredients. You simply begin by chopping, powdering, crushing, or grinding the herbal material as small as possible and place it in a skillet or a crock pot. Place enough lard or butter in the pan or pot to cover the herb. Leave the mixture over the very lowest heat for a while—at least ten to twenty minutes for a leafy substance, forty to sixty minutes for roots. Let the ointment cool, and store in the refrigerator. These traditional ointments, because they are made from perishable foods, don't keep very well. For a more permanent salve, use beeswax instead of lard or butter. Also, beeswax will stay solid at room temperature, so you don't need to refrigerate it.

Pond's family physician, a homeopathic doctor named Frederick Humphrey, M.D., obtained some of the medicine and tried it out. With his recommendation, its use soon spread rapidly among the other homeopaths of New York. Eventually the product's use spread even further amongst the medical profession. It became a popular over-the-counter remedy throughout the United States and in Europe. By the late 1880s it was a standard toiletry item in hotels in Paris and London. Pond's Extract Company survived into the 20th century. It is the source of the famous Pond's cold cream, which, in its original formula, also contained witch hazel extract.

Witch hazel bark contains astringent compounds that help shrink swollen tissues, although these are not the medicinal ingredients in the witch hazel extract sold in stores today. The bark also contains small amounts of the substance phenol, which escapes with the steam and is captured in the extraction process. Large amounts of phenol are poisonous, but tiny amounts can be used medicinally as a topical anesthetic, antiseptic, and anti-itching agent.

☞ DIRECTIONS: Purchase some witch hazel extract at a pharmacy. Moisten toilet paper and apply to painful or itching hemorrhoids every time you go to the bathroom.

CHAMOMILE OR YARROW TEA: Chamomile tea *(Matricaria recutita, Anthemis nobilis),* applied directly to the hemorrhoids, is a treatment from German folk medicine. Chamomile contains strong anti-inflammatory substances that may reduce the pain or itching of hemorrhoids. Yarrow tea *(Achillea millefolium)* may also do the trick: Yarrow contains some of the same anti-inflammatory constituents as chamomile.

☞ DIRECTIONS: Make enough strong chamomile or yarrow tea to use in a sitz bath. (Use 1 ounce of either herb for every 2 quarts of water.) Put the hot tea in a bucket or tub just big enough to sit in. There should be enough tea in the bucket to cover the hemorrhoids. Soak in the tea for fifteen minutes, two to three times a day, for an acute hemorrhoid attack. Alternately, you can make a quart of the tea and apply it hot to the hemorrhoids with a cotton cloth each time you use the bathroom.

HORSE CHESTNUTS: Indiana folklore suggests soothing hemorrhoid pain with an ointment made from horse chestnuts *(Aesculus hippocastanum),* also called buckeyes. Horse chestnut extracts are used in European conventional medicine for hemorrhoids and varicose veins. These extracts, which contain standardized amounts of aescin, are available in some United States health food stores. The constituent aescin tightens swollen veins.

☞ DIRECTIONS: Split six buckeyes, remove the shells, and chop up the contents as small as possible. Place in a skillet, cover with lard, and simmer for an hour. Allow to

Mild Laxatives

Conventional doctors recommend the use of mild laxatives to treat constipation that often accompanies hemorrhoids. Mild laxatives also appear widely in folk medicine as internal treatments to accompany the various external remedies for hemorrhoids. It is important not to use strong stimulating laxatives when suffering from hemorrhoids because these laxatives can irritate the inflamed tissues. The mild laxatives burdock root (*Arctium lappa*), dandelion root (*Taraxacum officinale*), psyllium seed (*Plantago spp.*), and yellow dock (*Rumex crispus*) are recommended and appear in this section.

cool until the ointment is solid. Apply to the hemorrhoids several times a day. Alternately, you can look for ready-made horse chestnut ointments at your health food store or herb shop.

CALENDULA: The Amish suggest using an ointment of calendula flowers (*Calendula officinalis*) to treat hemorrhoids. Calendula, which is also called pot marigold, is a different plant from garden marigolds (*Tagetes erecta*) and it contains different constituents. Calendula contains anesthetic and anti-inflammatory constituents as well as other constituents that promote the healing of wounds. Calendula-based ointments made with beeswax are available in health food stores and herb shops and are often combined with other herbs.

☞ DIRECTIONS: Purchase a commercial calendula ointment at a health food store or herb shop and apply to the hemorrhoids each time you use the bathroom.

ALOE VERA: Aloe vera is best known as a pain-relieving remedy for mild burns. But it may also be effective for the pain and itching of hemorrhoids. The same anti-inflammatory constituents that reduce blistering and inflammation in burns

Garlic Clove

Several folk sources mention the practice of inserting a peeled garlic clove into the anus to treat hemorrhoids. This method is also mentioned in some contemporary herbal texts. But it's best to avoid this method, because raw garlic can cause skin burns, including serious second- and third-degree burns. The area just inside the anus has no nerve endings, so you could burn your rectum with the garlic and not even realize it. Garlic should never be left on the skin for more than 20 to 30 minutes at a time.

may also reduce the irritation of hemorrhoids.

☞ DIRECTIONS: Break off a piece of an aloe vera leaf. Apply the clear mucilage (and not the yellow sap under the leaf) to the hemorrhoids each time you use the bathroom. Alternately, you can purchase aloe vera gel at a health food store or drugstore.

RED CLOVER: A salve made from red clover blossoms is a hemorrhoid remedy from the Amish and also from the folk medicine of New England. The blossoms of red clover, like mullein leaf above, contain the topical anti-inflammatory constituent coumarin. The clover blossoms also contain a variety of other aromatic anti-inflammatory constituents.

☞ DIRECTIONS: Chop ½ ounce of red clover blossoms and spread on the bottom of a skillet. Add enough lard to cover. Apply just enough heat to melt the lard, and stir the clover blossoms into the lard. Remove from the heat and allow to stand until the salve becomes solid. Apply to the hemorrhoids each time you use the bathroom.

OINTMENT FORMULA—GREASE ONESELF: An ointment for hemorrhoids that combines several other herbs in this section was suggested by a Mr. P. Smith in 1812, according to Clarence Meyer's *American Folk Medicine.* The remedy is slightly modified here to include only the plants that are likely to be available for purchase in stores today.

☞ DIRECTIONS: Take one handful each of plantain leaf, burdock root, and mullein leaf. Powder the roots in a coffee grinder, and crumble the leaves. Place all the items in a skillet, and add a pound of butter. Melt the butter, and simmer on the lowest heat for thirty to forty minutes. Remove from the heat and let cool to room temperature. Place in another container and put in the refrigerator until the butter is solid. "Grease oneself," said Smith.

DANDELION ROOT TEA: Dandelion root tea (*Taraxacum officinale*) is sometimes used in the folk medicine of Hispanics in the Southwest as a laxative for constipation accompanying hemorrhoids. The root stimulates the flow of bile, which in turn promotes normal elimination. As a laxative, dandelion root is very mild, making it appropriate for use with hemorrhoids. Dandelion is approved in Germany as a digestive aid and liver stimulant. Don't take dandelion root if you have gallstones or pain and inflammation in the digestive tract, however.

☞ DIRECTIONS: Place 1 ounce of dandelion root in 1 quart of water. Cover the pot, bring the water to a boil, and then simmer on the lowest heat for forty minutes. Remove from heat and let cool to room temperature. Drink the quart of tea in 3 or 4 doses during the day. Continue for up to three weeks.

BURDOCK ROOT: Burdock root (*Arctium lappa*), along with dandelion root, is one of the top ten herbs prescribed by North American professional medical herbalists today. Burdock is mild in its actions, and herbalists consider it to be the best choice when mild actions are preferred, as in the case of constipation accompanying hemorrhoids. Burdock increases the flow of bile from the liver and has mild laxative and diuretic effects. It also gently increases the blood circulation to the skin and, presumably, to the swollen hemorrhoids. When taken as a tea, burdock's complex carbohydrate constituents may also feed the "friendly" bacteria in the bowels, helping to restore balance and correct constipation due to any bacteria imbalances.

☞ DIRECTIONS: Place 1 ounce of burdock root in 1 quart of water. Cover the pot, bring the water to a boil, and then simmer on the lowest heat for forty minutes. Remove from heat and let cool to room temperature. Drink the quart of tea in 3 or 4 doses during the day for three weeks.

CARROT BOLUS: A hemorrhoid remedy from New England calls for a grated carrot bolus. This bolus is a herbal preparation that is inserted into the anus to treat protruding hemorrhoids. The pressure of the grated carrot bolus works by pressing the hemorrhoids back into the tissue surrounding the rectum. The carrot is grated and used for its firm texture.

☞ DIRECTIONS: Grate a small carrot. Mix it with enough lard to hold the soft mass together. Insert the bolus into the anus and hold it in place as long as possible.

PSYLLIUM SEED: According to Hispanic folklore of the American Southwest, psyllium seed (*Plantago spp.*) is recommended as a bulk laxative for bleeding hemorrhoids. Psyllium seed is beneficial for bleeding hemorrhoids because it softens the stool, reducing the irritation and pressure on the swollen veins. Today, conventional doctors throughout the United States recommend psyllium-based laxatives for constipation accompanying hemorrhoids.

☞ DIRECTIONS: For bleeding hemorrhoids, purchase a psyllium-based laxative at a pharmacy, supermarket, or health food store. Follow the instructions on the label.

ONIONS: Several North American folk sources suggest eating onions for hemorrhoids. In their book *Home Remedies: Hydrotherapy, Massage, Charcoal, and Other Simple Treatments*, Agatha Thrash, M.D.,

FOLK REMEDIES

and Calvin Thrash, M.D., physicians who are affiliated with the Seventh Day Adventist religion, recommend eating cooked onions to stop the bleeding of hemorrhoids. Russian folklore calls for steaming the hemorrhoids with the fumes of cooked onions. It is conceivable that anti-inflammatory compounds in cooked onions could actually reduce the inflammation and itching of hemorrhoids.

☞ DIRECTIONS: Place 4 large onions, peeled and chopped, into a half gallon of milk in a large pot. Cover and heat the mixture in an oven on low heat. Remove the pot from the oven, remove the lid, and cover with a toilet seat. Take a seat and let the onion fumes steam the hemorrhoids. (Be very careful not to burn yourself on the hot pot.) Complete the treatment by applying Vaseline to the hemorrhoids.

HEAT AND STEAM: New England residents report that the application of

heat, in the form of steam, hot baths, or other hot applications, can relieve the discomfort of hemorrhoids. The Seventh Day Adventists recommend taking a hot sitz bath for hemorrhoid pain. Conventional physicians say the same. The physiological action of the hot water increases circulation in the veins around the anus, removing the stagnancy of blood that contributes to the swelling and discomfort of hemorrhoids.

☞ DIRECTIONS: Run enough hot water in a tub to cover the hips when seated. For acute hemorrhoids, sit in the tub with your feet out of the water for ten to fifteen minutes twice a day.

COLD BATH: At the turn of the century, German immigrants, who arrived here with their own system of folk water cures, recommended treating hemorrhoids with cold sitz baths instead of hot ones. The cold baths are indicated, according to the Germans, between acute

232

attacks—not when there is active pain, inflammation, or swelling in the hemorrhoids. The baths work by constricting the blood vessels of the hemorrhoids.

☞ DIRECTIONS: Run enough cold water in the bathtub to cover the hips when sitting. Between acute hemorrhoid attacks, sit in the tub with your feet out of the water, for forty seconds to two minutes, depending on your tolerance to the cold water. Do this in the evening before bed three times a week.

❦ Hiccups ❧

🔲 🔲 🔲

A hiccup is an involuntary spasm of the diaphragm followed by a sharp intake of air that is abruptly stopped by a sudden, involuntary closing of the glottis (an opening between the vocal cords). The consequent blocking of air produces the repeated sharp sound, which sounds like hic.

The cause of short episodes of hiccups is unknown. Episodes of prolonged or recurrent hiccups may be the result of swallowing hot or irritating substances, pneumonia, alcoholism, certain prescription drugs, disorders of the stomach, pregnancy, or even some emotional disorders.

According to conventional medicine, a high blood level of carbon dioxide inhibits hiccups. You can bring on a high blood level of carbon dioxide by holding your breath, a solution to hiccups that is used in many folk traditions. Modern medicine and folk medicine also suggest stimulating the vagus nerve, one of the nerves that activates the diaphragm, which can be done simply by swallowing.

Some serious illnesses can cause persistent hiccups, but the occasional passing episodes are no cause for concern. However, if your hiccups persist for longer than eight hours, or you suspect that a prescription drug may be causing your hiccups, give your doctor a call.

Remedies

GYPSY HICCUP CURE: A Gypsy folk tradition suggests drinking the following tea to cure hiccups. The herbs used in the tea have sedative, anti-inflammatory, and anti-spasmodic properties. Whether these properties have an actual effect on the nerves or muscles responsible for producing hiccups is not clear. In any case, it is a nutritious and relaxing tea.

☞ DIRECTIONS: Take a handful each of valerian root, blackberry leaf, fennel seeds, chamomile flowers, peppermint leaf, and sage leaf. Crush and mix well in a bowl. Place 2 tablespoons of the dried herbs in a 1-pint jar. Fill with boiling water and cover. Steep for ten to fifteen minutes. Strain and drink 1 cup of warm (not hot) tea three times a day for up to ten days.

LEMONADE: A North Carolina remedy for hiccups calls for taking nine swallows of lemonade. Another suggestion from the same state calls for nine sips of water. (Thus, it seems to be the repetition of swallowing, not the substance sipped, that's important.) Taking so many sips involves not only repeated gulping, but

Things to Swallow

According to conventional medicine, the simple action of swallowing can end a case of the hiccups. Swallowing stimulates the vagus nerve, one of the nerves that controls the diaphragm and other muscles involved in breathing. Folk traditions recommend a wide variety of things to swallow to cure hiccups, including: dill seeds, peanut butter, sugar, lemonade, strong coffee, water, crushed ice, and cold soda water. It is not clear whether it's the substance that is swallowed or the action of swallowing that is responsible for the remedy's benefits.

it requires holding the breath for a while—both of which are conventional mechanisms for stopping hiccups.

☞ DIRECTIONS: To cure hiccups, make some lemonade and take 9 consecutive sips.

DILL SEED: Several entries in folklorist Clarence Meyer's *American Folk Medicine* suggest taking dill seeds (*Anethum graveolens*) to cure hiccups. The same treatment is mentioned in contemporary Indiana folklore. How the remedy works is not clear. It may be that

some properties of the seeds are at work, or that the difficulty in swallowing them stimulates the vagus nerve to terminate the hiccups.

☞ DIRECTIONS: Chew and swallow a teaspoon of dill seeds.

SUGAR OR HONEY: Eating sugar or honey is one of the most widespread folk cures for hiccups. The ancient Aztecs recommended swallowing honey; this same practice persists today in the folk traditions of Mexico and the American Southwest. A spoonful of sugar is preferred in North Carolina and Indiana folklore. Both substances are difficult to swallow, which may stimulate the vagus nerve and help stop the hiccups.

☞ DIRECTIONS: Take 1 teaspoonful of dry sugar into the mouth and swallow it. Or, swallow 1 tablespoon of honey.

HOLD UP: A North Carolina hiccup remedy recommends holding your arm above your head. This action may change the tension in the muscles used in breathing, thus breaking the rhythm of the hiccups. The posture may also stimulate the vagus nerve, which descends through the muscles that connect the neck to the shoulder.

☞ DIRECTIONS: Hold your arms over your head and shake them. It may help to hold your breath as long as possible while doing so.

Water Cures

Drinking water is a universal remedy for hiccups, mentioned not only in conventional medicine, but also in folk traditions throughout North America. The variations of this remedy are plentiful: Sip water without taking a breath. Drink a glass of water while holding the nose. Drink as many swallows of water as you can without taking a breath. Block the ears with one finger from each hand while taking five sips of water from a glass on a table. (The number of sips varies from tradition to tradition—five, seven, eight, or nine sips are all cited.) Drink a cupful of cold water in nine gulps. Drink cold soda water instead of tap water.

Interestingly, you don't always have to drink the water to cure yourself of hiccups. According to one North Carolina remedy, simply staring into a glass of water is enough to cure you of the affliction!

HOLD YOUR BREATH: In his collection of folk cures called *American Folk Medicine,* folklorist Clarence Meyer calls for simply holding your breath. This remedy is also recommended in conventional medicine, because holding the breath increases the carbon dioxide level in the blood, which helps to end the hiccups. This method is also mentioned in the folklore of New England, Indiana, and Kentucky.

☞ DIRECTIONS: Hold the breath as long as possible. Repeat until the hiccups are cured.

BOO!: Scaring someone with the hiccups is a well-known cure. This remedy's benefit may be due to the person's suddenly inhaling and holding his breath. A remedy used in Kentucky folk medicine suggests surprising the sufferer by suddenly popping a paper bag behind him.

☞ DIRECTIONS: Find some suitable—but safe—way to surprise the sufferer.

THUMBS BEHIND THE EARS: A remedy from North Carolina suggests placing the tips of the thumbs behind your ears and pushing inward on the skull bones. This region behind the ears is where the vagus nerve exits the skull and descends toward the respiratory muscles. So pressure in that area may actually have a physiological effect on the respiratory system.

☞ DIRECTIONS: Place the thumbs behind the ears and press inward until hiccups subside.

THINK OF THE ONE YOU LOVE: Possibly the most pleasant of the folk hiccup cures, practiced by individuals in both Indiana and North Carolina, is to think about the person you love the most. The North Carolina version of the remedy claims that if the person you love loves you back, the hiccups will stop.

☞ DIRECTIONS: Focus on the one you love.

❧ Indigestion and ❧ Heartburn

❋ ❋ ❋

Painful indigestion and heartburn are so common in the United States today that antacids are among the top-selling categories of over-the-counter drugs. This section deals specifically with digestive pain rather than sluggish, inefficient digestion. Although the two conditions may occur simultaneously, different folk remedies are usually prescribed for each. For instance, bitter herbs are commonly prescribed for sluggish digestion, but they are contraindicated if pain is present. Bitter herbs increase the secretion of digestive juices, which can increase pain (see "Digestion," page 162).

Simple digestive pain can come from two main causes: inflammation of the wall of the stomach or intestine, or spasms of the intestinal muscles, often in response to a buildup of gas. The most common causes of digestive inflammation are irritation of the digestive lining by the body's own digestive secretions, infection by a bacterium known as *Helicobacter pylori,* or irritation by offending foods. Persistent indigestion pain should be a cue to visit the doctor, who will help you experiment with your diet to determine and remove the cause.

Heartburn—a gassy, burning sensation in your upper abdomen, sometimes accompanied by the regurgitation of sour, bitter material into your throat or mouth—actually has nothing to do with your heart. Heartburn indicates that the lower part of your esophagus, the upper part of your stomach, or the first section of your bowel has become irritated, and the contents of your stomach have started to back up into the esophagus. Most cases of heartburn aren't serious. The easiest way to avoid a simple case of heartburn? Moderation. Heartburn is generally the result of eating too much too fast.

Eating while under stress is also a major cause of indigestion and heartburn. When relaxed, the body secretes its own antacids from the pancreas and bile ducts in response to food entering the intestine. In a state of stress, these secretions shut off. Thus "acid" indigestion may not be due to excess acid, but to a deficiency of the neutralizing secretions. The best way to turn these secretions back on is to relax for at least ten minutes before eating. Persistent inflammation of the digestive tract can cause ulceration. Ulcers can have serious and even fatal complications if they bleed or if the ulcer eats entirely through the intestine.

The most common categories of folk remedies for digestive pain and heartburn are demulcent herbs (slimy mucilaginous plants that coat and soothe inflamed tissue), herbs containing anti-inflammatory substances, and carminative herbs, which reduce the spasms of intestinal cramps that often accompany gas.

Remedies

SLIPPERY ELM: Slippery elm bark (*Ulmus fulva*) is used in modern European and North American professional medical herbalism as a soothing treatment for gastritis and ulcers of the digestive tract. The bark, when mixed with water, makes a slimy mucilaginous mass that is soothing to inflamed tissues. Please note that ulcers can cause internal bleeding and have serious health consequences. If you suffer from ulcers, be sure to see a doctor.

☞ DIRECTIONS: Place 1 tablespoon of powdered slippery elm bark in a cup. Fill with boiling water. Let steep for ten minutes. Stir, without straining, and drink the whole cup. Do this as needed for pain.

GINGER: Ginger (*Zingiber officinalis*) is a near-universal remedy for pain in the digestive tract, appearing in the folklore of New England, North Carolina, the southern Appalachians, Indiana, the Southwest, and China. The plant contains both antispasmodic and anti-inflammatory constituents. It also contains topical anesthetic compounds that may directly reduce pain in the digestive tract. In clinical trials ginger has shown to be effective in treating some kinds of nausea.

☞ DIRECTIONS: Thinly slice a fresh ginger root. (The root should be about the size of your thumb.) Place the slices in 1 quart of water. Bring to a boil, and then simmer on the lowest possible heat for thirty minutes in a covered pot. Let cool for thirty minutes more. Strain and drink ½ to 1 cup, sweetened with honey as desired.

If you don't have fresh ginger, stir ½ teaspoon of ground ginger into 1 cup of hot water. Let stand for two to three minutes. Strain and drink, as desired.

FENNEL: Today, in the professional medical herbalism of Great Britain,

Baking Soda

A do-it-yourself antacid remedy of questionable safety from various streams of North American folklore is to ingest baking soda. Habitual consumption of large amounts of baking soda can cause salt imbalances in the body, however. A safer method is to use commercial antacids, which contain measured amounts of bicarbonate and provide instructions for safe use on the label.

North America, and New Zealand, fennel *(Foeniculum vulgare)* is a commonly prescribed herb for abdominal cramping and gas in adults. It appears in the folk medicine of both New England and China. Fennel is an approved medicine in Germany for mild gastrointestinal complaints. It contains at least 16 chemical constituents with antispasmodic properties.

☞ DIRECTIONS: Crush 1 teaspoon of fennel seeds with a mortar and pestle or grind them in a coffee grinder. Place the cracked seeds in a cup and fill with boiling water. Cover and let sit for ten minutes. Strain and drink 3 cups of the warm tea each day on an empty stomach. Do this as often as desired.

CATNIP: Catnip is a widespread folk medicine for intestinal cramping and colic. It is included in the folk literature of New England, Appalachia, North Carolina, Indiana, and New Mexico. It is used by blacks throughout the deep South and by Hispanics in the Los Angeles area. Like chamomile, above, catnip contains both antispasmodic and sedative constituents. It was an official medicine in the *United States Pharmacopoeia* from 1840 until 1870.

☞ DIRECTIONS: Place 1 teaspoon of the dried herb in a cup and add boiling water. Cover and let stand for ten minutes. Strain and drink 3 cups a day, on an empty stomach, before meals. Do this as often as desired.

CARAWAY SEEDS: North Americans know caraway seeds *(Carum carvi)* as the tiny seeds coating the crust of rye bread. Caraway seeds are known throughout the Arabic world and in European folk medicine as a treatment for painful intestinal gas. The German government has approved caraway as an official medicine for that condition. The seeds are used for the same purpose in the folk medicine of North Carolina, Appalachia, and Indiana.

☞ DIRECTIONS: Place 1 teaspoon of crushed caraway seeds in a cup and add boiling water. Cover the cup and let stand for ten minutes. Strain and drink 3 cups of warm tea a day on an empty stomach. Alternately, you can simply chew on the seeds. Do this as often as desired.

FORMULA: The following formula, from contemporary North American professional medical herbalism, combines four of the remedies in this section.

☞ DIRECTIONS: Place 1 tablespoon each of chamomile flowers, mint leaves, fennel seeds, and slippery elm bark in a 1-pint jar. Fill the jar with boiling water and cover. Let stand until the water reaches room temperature, shaking the bottle occasionally to mix its con-

tents. Strain and drink the quart during the course of the day (on an empty stomach) between meals. Do this as often as desired.

CHAMOMILE: Chamomile *(Matricaria recutita, Anthemis nobilis)* is a popular folk remedy for treating stomachaches in New England, Indiana, and the Southwest. It is an approved medicine for this purpose in Germany. Chamomile contains at least 19 antispasmodic constituents as well as 5 sedative ones. A 1993 clinical trial showed that the plant was effective in relieving infant colic as well.

☞ DIRECTIONS: Place 1 tablespoon of chamomile flowers in a cup and add boiling water. Cover the cup and let stand for ten minutes. Strain and drink warm three times a day on an empty stomach. Do this for two to three weeks, and then take a break for a week or two. Note: In general, chamomile poses no health threat. If you have suffered previous anaphylactic shock reactions from ragweed, however, talk to your doctor before using this herb.

MINTS: Different types of mints, including peppermint and spearmint, are recommended for indigestion in the folk literature of New England, New York, North Carolina, Appalachia, Indiana, New Mexico, and California. Mints have also been used as carminatives by members of at least seven major North American Indian tribes. Mint is an official digestive aid in German medicine. Peppermint contains antispasmodic compounds. (It is better suited to treating abdominal cramping than heartburn. It can sometimes make heartburn worse.)

☞ DIRECTIONS: Place 1 teaspoon of the dried herb in a cup and add boiling water. Cover the cup and let steep for ten minutes. Strain well and drink 1 cup three times a day on an empty stomach. Do this as often as desired.

❦ Insomnia ❦

◼ ◼ ◼

At some point in our lives, between one third and one half of all Americans have a serious bout of chronic insomnia, which is the inability to sleep the desired amount at least three nights a week for a month or more. Insomnia may mean difficulty falling asleep, waking up periodically during the night, or waking up too early. Length of sleep is not a measure of insomnia, because different people require different amounts. So, if disturbed sleep leaves you feeling fatigued and not up to par the next day, you may be suffering from insomnia, even if you slept for eight hours. Brief spells of insomnia may accompany worry, stress, changes in job shifts, or other temporary life situations. Habitual coffee drinking, even if only a few cups a day, may also cause or contribute to insomnia. Chronic insomnia may accompany such conditions as depression; chronic pain; withdrawal from nicotine, alcohol, drugs, or sleep medications; or life passages such as menopause. Because some of these conditions become more prevalent as we age, insomnia is common among the elderly.

Insomnia can be the first sign of nutritional deficiencies, appearing before more serious diseases arise. It may indicate a deficiency of the minerals calcium, magnesium, or potassium, all of which are common deficiencies in the American diet. Deficiencies of the B-vitamins (niacin, pathothenic acid,

folic acid, biotin, and pyridoxine) or of vitamin E may also cause insomnia.

Chronic stress can also lead to insomnia. Our body possesses hormonal mechanisms to respond to brief periods of stress throughout the day. At night, our body is given a break from these mechanisms to recuperate. When the body adapts to persistent stress, however, we end up physically prepared to run from a bear, even at bedtime when we should be resting. Many of the folk remedies in this section help send cues to the brain, body, and glandular system that we are safe and that it is now time to relax and recuperate in order to meet the challenges of tomorrow.

Conventional medical treatment for chronic insomnia includes drugs in the benzodiazepine class, such as Valium and Xanax. These drugs may be appropriate to induce sleep during a brief crisis, but withdrawal from them may worsen the insomnia or induce anxiety, and use for as little as six weeks may cause addiction. These drugs, as well as over-the-counter sleep medications, can also disrupt patterns of sleep, interfering with the deepest stage of sleep known as deep delta wave sleep. During this part of sleep, the body normally recovers from stress, rebuilds its immune system, and repairs tissues. Chronic drug use can result in a constant feeling of fatigue, however. Before you turn to prescription or over-the-counter medications, you may want to try one of the folk remedies below for a healthier, more natural snooze.

Remedies

REACTIVE HYDROTHERAPY: As the name implies, hydrotherapy is therapy with water in any of its forms—ice, cold water, hot water, steam, freshwater, or water imbued with special minerals. Reactive hydrotherapy uses cool water treatments to provoke an increase in circulation in a certain area.

Cold initially drives blood out of an area, but eventually the body reacts by flooding the area with blood to warm it up. In Clarence Meyer's *American Folk Medicine* it is noted that reactive hydrotherapy will often "Soothe the wary brain, and quiet the nerves better than an opiate." Some forms of insomnia are accompanied by excess circulation to the brain, such as might accompany mental stress. A cool compress on the neck draws blood away from the brain, helping to soothe the mind.

☞ DIRECTIONS: Put a cloth soaked in cold water on the back of the neck, and cover it with a warm towel. Keep the cloth in place for no more than fifteen minutes.

HOT FOOT BATH: Another Seventh Day Adventist water treatment is the hot foot bath. The treatment draws blood away from the brain and upper body toward the feet. This is also a treatment for

Water Cures for Insomniacs

Water cures were widely used to treat insomnia and many other ailments in 19th century America. Such treatments eventually became institutionalized at health spas throughout the country. In Germany and France today, these treatments are considered part of conventional medicine—a patient may receive prescriptions, paid for by insurance, to spend up to three weeks resting and receiving daily hydrotherapy sessions at a spa. Treatments for insomnia include applications of hot, cold, or neutral-temperature water. You will need to experiment to find the water temperature that helps you get to sleep, however, because different people and different types of insomnia require different treatments. In general, very hot or very cold treatments tend to stimulate rather than sedate, so it's best to use moderate temperatures.

headaches due to congestion and menstrual cramps, so it may be especially helpful for insomnia that accompanies those conditions. You can add crushed mustard seeds to the water to increase the heating effect. Be sure to wrap the upper body in a blanket to avoid chills and promote sweating. You can also cover the head with a cloth soaked in cool water to decrease circulation to the brain. (Caution: People with insulin-dependent diabetes should not use this treatment due to the possibility of burning the feet.)

☞ DIRECTIONS: Soak the feet in hot water. The water should be moderately hot, but not so hot that you pull back from it. Continue soaking for about fifteen minutes before bedtime.

COLD HIP BATH: A hydrotherapy treatment used to treat insomnia by German immigrants of the late

19th and early 20th centuries was the cold hip bath. The body reacts to a short, cold stimulus by pulling blood away from the brain toward the site of the stimulus. The treatment is still recommended today by some naturopathic physicians. It has not been tested in formal scientific trials.

☞ DIRECTIONS: Sit in a tub filled with cool, but not extremely cold, water. The water level should reach just above your navel. Rest your feet on the edge of the tub so the water just covers your hips and abdomen. This position may be easier to negotiate in a large bucket or laundry tub. (If you do this, place the bucket or laundry tub in the bathtub to catch any water that spills when you get in.) Soak for forty seconds to two minutes before going to bed.

HOT FOMENTATION: An alternate treatment from the Seventh Day Adventists, a 150-year-old religious group that has long influenced folk medicine throughout North America, is to apply hot water to the back. In contrast to reactive hydrotherapy, this method uses heat to draw blood to the area.

☞ DIRECTIONS: Soak a cloth in moderately hot water and rest it on the spine for twenty to thirty minutes before bedtime.

ROSE OIL: An aromatic remedy from the Amish is to apply diluted rose oil to the forehead. The pleasant fragrance somehow tricks the brain into relaxing the body. Apply and leave on throughout the night.

☞ DIRECTIONS: Place 8 to 10 drops of concentrated rose oil in 1 ounce of almond oil. Apply a small amount to the forehead before going to bed.

THE NEUTRAL BATH: A standard Seventh Day Adventist water treatment for insomnia and nervous exhaustion is the neutral bath. Scientific studies have shown that taking a full immersion bath quiets *continued on page 251*

Soul Loss and Lost Souls

Soul loss. To many people in North America the loss of one's soul occurs at death. To others, soul loss is a crisis that leads to an illness that may ultimately result in debility or death. Medical anthropologists refer to soul loss as a "folk illness." Most of the illnesses treated in folk medicine are well known to doctors—from whooping cough to rabies, from burns to colds. From the medical viewpoint, some of the terms used in folk medicine to describe a condition are not quite right, even though the illnesses are recognizable. For example, in folk medicine, osteoarthritis and rheumatoid arthritis and a host of other achy, stiff conditions are all classified as rheumatism.

Some illnesses that are described in folk tradition are unknown to modern medicine. In fact, a case of soul loss may be mistaken for a contemporary disease, or doctors may believe that it is a sign of distress somehow caused by the culture in which the patient lives. However, it is always possible in such a case that folk knowledge may actually be ahead of medical knowledge, that a folk illness may be a real illness not yet recognized by medicine. This seems especially likely when the same illness is found in many different cultures—including some where it is not widely recognized. This is the case with soul loss.

Although it is found in many cultural groups in America, probably the best known example of American soul loss is in the Latino culture, where soul loss is called *susto,* meaning fright or trauma. The person suffering from susto is said to be restless in his sleep, and when he is awake he acts depressed, passive, or indifferent. Often the individual's grooming habits and cleanliness suffer. The illness is said to be caused by a sudden shock or fright that causes a person's soul to come loose and wander away or even be captured by a spirit. A typical situation leading to susto was described by a young Mexican woman who saw her father swept off his feet while fording a rapidly moving stream. He barely managed to save himself. Two weeks later she became ill and was diagnosed as suffering from susto.

In recent western European tradition, people are believed to have one soul. The soul is usually equated with consciousness. Therefore, you might expect a person whose soul has left him to appear unconscious. But, in many cultures, it is believed that humans have more than one soul. In such a tradition, one soul may be responsible for operating the basic functions of the body, such as breathing and heartbeat, and another for consciousness, since some activating principle obviously remains even when a person is unconscious. Still other cultures, for example the Hmong of southeast Asia, believe that a body has many souls.

Although the majority of Americans believe that humans have souls, and that their soul departs at death, there really is no "scientific proof" that souls really exist. How, then, can we approach the question of whether soul loss may represent folk knowledge that is beyond medical understanding? Investigating the beliefs and experiences of those who believe in soul loss will not help, because their beliefs may actually be producing the events and behaviors that define soul loss. However, we can study the possibility that soul loss traditions are valid by looking at cultures that do not have beliefs about soul loss and seeing whether the same experiences occur there. If the experiences do turn up in such nontraditional settings, then the idea of soul loss is valid.

Since Raymond Moody's book, *Life After Life,* appeared in 1974, the American public has shown a great deal of interest in one particular kind of soul loss experience—

the near-death experience (NDE). In the classic NDE, as described by Moody and many others since 1974, the subject is unconscious while their conscious soul moves around the environment. But that is not the only way that people experience NDEs. Sometimes, after a classic NDE, when the person's viewpoint returns to normal and he can again speak and walk, something feels like it has remained outside the body. One woman, whose experience occurred as a result of a bad reaction to medicine, claimed it felt as though the "real" her remained up by the ceiling in the spot from where she had observed her resuscitation. The sensation of being separated continued for two weeks and only ended when she had a vision of deceased relatives and friends who asked her to choose between life and death. She chose to live because of unfinished personal business. This is a common scenario in NDEs.

The following morning when the woman awoke, she said she felt as though her spirit, which had been trailing along behind her like a balloon on a string, was now back inside her. Before her spirit reentered her, she had been conscious but passive and indifferent to her surroundings. To others she had seemed depressed, though she did not recall feeling sad. She made a good recovery and returned to her daily activities. This woman's strange experience had been precipitated by a shock—a shock that occurred as a result of a reaction to medication. Her symptoms were the same as those reported from cultures where soul loss is recognized. Had she been in such a culture, she would have been diagnosed as susto.

There are several kinds of NDEs, although only a few are routinely publicized. It seems that people experience the sensation of self leaving the body in a variety of ways, and some of these are included in the folk illness category of soul loss. This is an instance in which folk medical traditions may have knowledge of an important human state that is virtually unknown to modern biomedicine.

the production of the "fight-or-flight" hormones from the adrenal glands. Thus, this treatment is proven to relax you when you're all wound up.

☞ DIRECTIONS: Fill the tub with water at or just below body temperature, about 94–98°F. Soak for as long as one hour before bedtime.

HERBAL BATHS: Herbal baths were popular among German immigrants, and they remain popular in Germany today. When you bathe with herbs, your skin absorbs their essential oils. An herb's aroma may also help to induce a peaceful state of mind. You can add relaxing herbs to any of the baths previously described. Avoid using oils such as peppermint, clove, and cinnamon, however. These hot oils can burn sensitive skin.

☞ DIRECTIONS: Place 1 ounce of valerian, hop, chamomile, or lavender in a pot and cover with 1 quart of boiling water. Strain and add the water to the bath. Another ap-

proach is to add 1 or 2 drops of essential oil to the tub water. Remember that herbal oils are highly concentrated, so a little goes a long way. Enjoy an herbal bath right before bedtime.

DILL SEEDS: A folk remedy from China is to wash the head in a tea of dill seeds *(Anethum graveolens)* so you'll inhale the fumes of the tea. Dill contains a number of sedative constituents in its volatile oil, which may explain the value of the plant for insomnia. Dill itself has not been tested by scientists for these purposes.

☞ DIRECTIONS: If you don't want to smell like a pickle all night, here's a modified version of this remedy: Put 8 to 10 drops of essential oil of dill in 1 ounce of another oil, such as almond oil. Apply the mixture to a cloth, and keep it near your nose while you sleep. No direct application to the head is necessary. To avoid burns and blisters, never apply an essential oil in its con-

Valerian

Valerian is one of the most famous herbs for treating insomnia; it is still used today in folk remedies in New England, Appalachia, and Indiana. Scientific studies show that, for some people, it is as effective as the drug Valium in inducing sleep. It doesn't work for everyone, however, and can actually produce insomnia in some people.

United States physicians of the last century listed valerian as a sedative, but also called it a cerebral stimulant, which means it increases the blood flow to the brain. Herbal texts of the time recommended it for restless individuals with cold constitutions (those with a pale face, cold hands and feet, and a desire for warm drinks and extra layers of clothes). It was not recommended for "hot-headed" individuals (those with a red, flushed face and a desire for cold drinks and fewer layers of clothes). Today, valerian is usually combined with another herb such as hop to avoid the occasional stimulating effects of valerian.

centrated form directly to the skin.

PINE, JUNIPER, AND SAGE: A very common American Indian aromatherapy technique to induce sleep uses the scents of pine *(Pinus spp.)*, juniper *(Juniperus spp.)*, or sage *(Artemesia spp., Salvia spp.)*. The remedy requires burning and then inhaling the fresh or dried needles or leaves of the herbs. Also, you can inhale the scent by pouring a tea made from the dried plant over hot rocks.

☞ DIRECTIONS: You can adapt this technique for household use by burning the dried needles or leaves like incense. Take some dried needles or leaves of pine, juniper, or sage, light them with a match, blow the flame out, and put the smoking embers in an ashtray. Inhale the fragrance as it fills the room.

THE HOP PILLOW: A widespread folk cure for insomnia is the hop pillow. Hop *(Humulus lupulus)* has been used for centuries as a mild sedative. German and British immigrants, Seventh Day Adventists, Indiana farmers, and residents of the American Southwest have all used hop to help induce sleep. Hop was listed as an official medicine in the *United States Pharmacopoeia* from 1820 to 1926.

☞ DIRECTIONS: Cut two 8×11-inch squares of muslin fabric. Place 1 muslin square on top of the other and pin together around the edges. Sew ½-inch seams along the two long sides and one short side of the fabric, leaving the second short side open. Turn the seams to the inside. Take 4 ounces of hop, the fresher the better. Sprinkle it with a small amount of alcohol to bring out the active principle, but not enough to make it soggy. Add the herb to the muslin pillow case. Spread the herbs evenly within the pillow. (You will place it in your bed pillow, so you don't want it to make a lump.) Turn the raw edges under and pin the opening shut to enclose the content of the pillow securely.

Hop can also be used to make a soothing tea. Place 1 tablespoon of the herb in a cup and cover with boiling water. Cover the cup and let stand for ten minutes. Strain and drink before bedtime.

EXERCISE: According to the Seventh Day Adventists, the best way to put yourself to sleep is to make yourself tired.

☞ DIRECTIONS: Get twenty to forty minutes of

proper moderate physical exercise each day. Try going for a brisk walk or participating in a sport or a hobby you enjoy.

MASSAGE: Another Seventh Day Adventist method to induce sleep is to give the person with insomnia a gentle stroking massage. Scientific research shows that massage can induce relaxation and ease stress.

☞ DIRECTIONS: Massage the patient gently, with the strokes always moving in the direction of the heart.

CATNIP: Catnip (*Napeta cataria*) tea has been a popular sleep aid in America since the arrival of the first European immigrants. The plant arrived with the colonists and became rapidly naturalized here. Indian tribes, including the Onondaga and Cayuga, used it to calm sleepless and peevish children.

The Seventh Day Adventists continue to use catnip today to induce sleep, and a 1995 poll of contempo-

rary professional herbalists concluded that catnip remains one of the most prescribed herbs for insomnia.

☞ DIRECTIONS: Place 1 to 3 teaspoons of the dried herb in a cup and cover with boiling water. Cover and let sit for ten minutes. Strain and drink before bedtime. When making the tea, contemporary Appalachian herbalist Tommie Bass suggests combining catnip with passion flower, sage, peppermint, or skullcap.

PASSION FLOWER: From the southern Appalachians to the American Southwest, people have long used passion flower (*Passiflora incarnata*) as a sedative to aid in sleep. The Amish combine it with chamomile. Passion flower contains sedative alkaloid constituents that help you relax.

☞ DIRECTIONS: Place a heaping teaspoon of passion flower in 1 cup of water and steep ten minutes. Strain and drink before retiring for the night.

Herbs for Insomnia

Today, medical herbalists often use plant medicines as minor sedatives. In general, herbs will not force you to sleep like some of the stronger pharmaceutical medicines used for the same purpose. Instead, herbs may gently trigger your innate sleep response. It is best to take them as warm teas, because warm fluid in the stomach also has a relaxing effect. Take a $1/2$-cup dose an hour before bedtime to help calm you, and then take a second dose just before going to bed. For severe insomnia, try adding a one-third dose just after dinner, and keep a fourth dose by the bed in case you awaken during the night. Sedative herbs may work better in combinations of three or more; different herbs help induce sleep through various mechanisms.

CHAMOMILE: Chamomile tea *(Matricaria recutita, Anthemis nobilis)* is one of the most popular commercial beverages used today to induce relaxation and sleep. The plant came to North America with the colonists and is now native to many areas of the country. It has been used in folk medicine in New England, Appalachia, the Midwest and Southwest, and possibly everywhere in between. Chamomile's constituents, which have both anti-inflammatory and antispasmodic actions, also promote digestion. It may be especially suited for insomnia that accompanies inflammation or digestive upset. (Note: Chamomile is not appropriate for habitual use because it may suppress normal and healthy inflammatory responses. Occasional use is safe, but don't use daily for more than two to three weeks. In addition, chamomile flowers may cause symptoms of allergies in some people allergic to ragweed and related plants, although the risk of this is quite low.)

☞ DIRECTIONS: Put a heaping tablespoon of chamomile flowers in a cup and add boiling water. Cover and steep for ten minutes. Strain and drink before turning in for the night.

HOT MILK: Drink a cup of hot milk before bedtime. This New England remedy has doubtlessly appeared wherever milk is consumed and persists today in the folk medicine of the United States. How does it work? The warm milk may trigger instincts of safety associated with nursing at the breast. Variations of this remedy include adding ½ teaspoon of nutmeg or 2 teaspoons of honey. (Note: Nutmeg has psychoactive constituents that can induce unpleasant hallucinations in doses of only several teaspoons.)

☞ DIRECTIONS: Warm the milk and drink before bedtime. It'll cultivate pleasant, relaxing thoughts.

DEEP BREATHING: Another Seventh Day Adventist technique is to take slow, deep breaths. Breathing techniques are used throughout the world to relax the body and slow the mind. Research into the breathing techniques of yoga shows that deep breathing actually changes the brain waves, inducing a more relaxed state.

☞ DIRECTIONS: Take 10 to 20 slow, deep breaths of fresh air at an open window or while lying in bed.

GINSENG WINE: For insomnia that results from chronic stress or an illness, especially a feverish illness, try making an herbal wine out of American ginseng (Panax quinquefolium)—not Asian ginseng. American ginseng in various forms is used in

Chinese folk medicine and throughout Chinatowns in North America today.

☞ DIRECTIONS: Chop 3½ ounces of American ginseng and place it in 1 quart of liquor such as vodka. Let the mixture stand for five to six weeks in a cool, dark place, turning the container frequently. Then take 1 ounce of the solution after dinner or before bed. (You don't need to strain the liquid in this remedy. The root is heavy and will settle at the bottom of the container.) Be sure to use American ginseng, not Asian ginseng, in this remedy.

❧ Itching and Rashes ❧

▨ ▨ ▨

An itch may be due to local irritation of the skin. Local irritation may be caused by insect bites, stings, or infestation; by an allergic reaction to a plant, animal, or synthetic substance; or by infection from molds, yeasts, or other microorganisms. Sometimes itching can be simply due to dry skin. Many prescription drugs can also cause itching.

An itch may also be due to a systemic disease—one that's irritating the skin from the inside out. For example, disorders of the blood, kidneys, or thyroid can cause itching. An itch from a systemic disease may affect only a small area of the skin, as in cases of eczema or psoriasis or allergies to substances that have been eaten. Sometimes a systemic disease will cause itching over large areas of the body or itching that moves from one place to another.

Conventional treatment of itching and rashes first requires an investigation of the cause of the skin condition. For example, if itching is the result of an allergic sensitivity to a certain fabric, avoiding that particular fabric is likely to be recommended. If prescription drugs are responsible for your discomfort, your physician may prescribe a different medication. Folk remedies traditionally rely on herbs to treat and soothe the skin. If your doctor has diagnosed your skin condition as one that can be self treated, you may want to try some of the remedies below.

Remedies

JUNIPER AND CLOVE: Folklorist Clarence Meyer's *American Folk Medicine* suggests using a salve of juniper *(Juniperus spp.)* and clove *(Eugenia carophyllata)* to soothe itchy skin. Juniper berries have been used to treat itching by American Indians of the Paiute, Shoshone, and Cherokee tribes. Clove has been used throughout Asia, the Middle East, Mexico, and the American Southwest to treat itchy skin conditions. Juniper contains anti-inflammatory volatile substances, and clove contains the substance eugenol, a topical anesthetic widely used by dentists. The eugenol presumably affects the itch by numbing the nerve endings in the skin. The following salve is modified slightly from the one in Meyer's collection.

☞ DIRECTIONS: Melt 3 ounces of unsalted butter in a sauce pan. Then, in a separate pan, melt a lump of beeswax about the size of 2 tablespoons (it is difficult to get beeswax actually into the tablespoon). When the beeswax is melted, add it to the melted butter and stir well. Add 5 tablespoons of ground juniper berries and 3 tablespoons of ground clove to the butter/beeswax mixture and stir. (Instead of purchasing the herbs as powders, it is best to grind the herbs yourself because the volatile substances are preserved better in the whole berries and clove.) Allow the mixture to cool and become solid. Apply as a salve to itchy skin.

MINT: Another remedy from Chinese folk medicine for treating itchy skin rashes or hives is a wash of mint tea. In China, cornmint *(Mentha arvensis)* is the type of mint used. In North America, peppermint *(Mentha piperita),* which has constituents similar to cornmint, is preferred. Both peppermint and cornmint contain significant amounts of menthol, which has anesthetic and anti-inflammatory properties when applied topically. In general, mint also contains high amounts of the anti-inflammatory rosmarinic acid, which is readily absorbed into the skin.

☞ DIRECTIONS: Place 1 ounce of dried peppermint leaves in a 1-pint jar and fill with boiling water. Immediately cover the jar to prevent the escape of the aromatic eugenol from the tea. Allow to cool to room temperature. Strain, dip a clean cloth in the tea, and apply to the itchy area as often as necessary.

BASIL: A wash of basil tea *(Ocimum basilicum)* is used in Chinese folk medicine to treat itching from hives. Basil, like cloves, contains high amounts of eugenol, a topical anesthetic.

☞ DIRECTIONS: Place ½ ounce of dried basil leaves in a 1-pint jar and fill with boiling water. Immediately cover to prevent the escape of the aromatic eugenol from the tea. Allow to cool to room temperature. Strain, dip a clean cloth in the tea, and apply to itchy areas as often as desired.

THYME: A remedy from Chinese folk medicine, similar to the two above, uses garden thyme *(Thymus vulgaris).* Thyme contains large amounts of the volatile constituent thymol, which gives thyme some of its fragrance. Thanks to thymol's anesthetic and anti-inflammatory properties, it numbs the nerves that cause the itch while reducing local inflammation. A Chinese tradition suggests mixing thyme with dandelion root.

☞ DIRECTIONS: Place 1 ounce of dried dandelion root and ½ ounce of dried thyme leaves in a 1-quart jar. Fill with boiling water and cover with a tight lid. Allow to cool to room temperature. Strain, dip a cloth in the tea, and apply to the affected areas.

CLEAVERS: Cleavers (*Galium aparine*) has been used to treat skin ailments since the time of the ancient Greeks. American Indians of the Iroquois and Chippewa tribes later used cleavers for the same purpose. Today, teas made from the plant remain a common prescription by professional herbalists in North America for treating skin ailments.

No constituents with specific anti-inflammatory or anti-itch properties have been identified in cleavers. Herbalists theorize that the constituents work by "purifying the blood"— that is, by treating the itch from the inside out. No scientific evidence for such an action is apparent, however. Its constituents include tannins, which may account for the mild astringent action it possesses. Dried cleavers is rich in mineral nutrition, with an ounce of the herb providing significant portions of the daily requirement of such minerals as calcium, magnesium, and iron.

☞ DIRECTIONS: Place 1 ounce of dried cleavers in a quart of water, and simmer for twenty minutes. Strain and drink as a beverage throughout the day. Sweeten with honey if desired. Drink 3 to 4 cups a day for two to three weeks and see if your skin condition improves.

LEMON JUICE: Rubbing lemon juice on itchy, inflamed skin is recommended in American folklorist Clarence Meyer's *American Folk Medicine*. The same method is used in the Hispanic folklore of the American Southwest. The aromatic substances in lemon have anesthetic and anti-inflammatory properties, which may be responsible for its medicinal activity, if any in fact exists.

☞ DIRECTIONS: Juice a lemon. Apply undiluted to itchy skin.

BAKING SODA BATH: A baking soda bath is recommended for itchy skin conditions in the Hispanic folklore of the Southwest. The same treatment is used in New England. Contemporary Seventh Day Adventists, a religious movement that advocates natural remedies and alternative medicine, also use baking soda baths for treating itchy skin conditions, eczema, and sunburn.

☞ DIRECTIONS: Add 1 cup of commercial baking soda to a tub of 94–98°F water. Stay in the tub for thirty to sixty minutes. Let the skin dry naturally without toweling.

PLANTAIN: Plantain *(Plantago major)* was called "Englishman's footprint" by the American Indians and by residents of the Southwest because the herb came to North America with the immigrants from the British Isles and rapidly spread to wherever the immigrants went. Today it can be found in lawns and along sidewalks throughout North America. Foot baths of "English" plantain are used in the folk medicine of northern New Mexico to alleviate itchy feet. Plantain teas are also recommended in the southern Appalachian mountains to treat itchy skin conditions. Plantain contains small amounts of at least 14 different anti-inflammatory constituents, which, acting together, might be responsible for its itch-reducing effects.

☞ DIRECTIONS: Place 1 ounce of dried plantain leaf in a 1-quart jar and fill with boiling water. Cover and let cool to room temperature. Strain and apply the tea with a clean cloth to the affected areas.

ALOE VERA: Aloe vera may be helpful for treating itchy skin as well as minor burns, according to the traditions of the Seventh Day Adventists, a religious movement that advocates natural remedies and alternative medicine. The plant's anti-inflammatory constituents that reduce blistering and inflammation in burns may also reduce itching (see "Burns and Sunburn," page 97). Avoid using yellowish sap under the aloe's green skin. This area of the plant contains antraquinones, which may irritate the skin or eyes.

☞ DIRECTIONS: Break off a leaf, slice it down the middle, and rub the gel on the skin. You can also apply store-bought aloe vera gel or juice.

An alternative formula involves using olive oil to extend the aloe vera sap. Here's how: Add 8 ounces of extra virgin olive oil to 2 ounces of freshly squeezed aloe vera sap. Place the sap in a large bowl and add the oil a few drops at a time, constantly stirring. Rub the mixture on the skin.

CLAY: The American Indians commonly applied muddy clay to itchy skin areas. Clay applications were also commonly used in German and French folk medicine. Today, the practice remains highly recommended by contemporary Seventh Day Adventists for soothing the skin.

☞ DIRECTIONS: For this remedy, you can use bentonite clay, French green clay, or other cosmetic clay—all of which are available in health food stores and cosmetic outlets. Mix clay into 1 cup of warm (not hot) water until it is the consistency of a thin pea soup. Apply it to the skin. Let the clay stay on for at least forty minutes, or for several hours, if possible. Wipe off the clay using water and a wash cloth. (You may need to scrub gently with the cloth to remove the clay if the clay has dried completely.) Wipe off the clay over a bowl and discard the waste in your garden or on your lawn because clay can stop up your pipes. Repeat as often as desired.

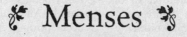 Menses

Menstruation is the monthly breakdown and discharge of portions of the endometrial tissue that lines the uterus. The normal menstrual cycle can vary from 21 to 35 days, with the flow lasting from 2 to 9 days. A 30 to 60 milliliter blood loss (1 to 2 ounces) is expected. Disorders of the cycle can be due to the length of the cycle, length (or lack of) menstrual flow, and the amount of the flow. Here are some medical terms and definitions for some abnormal menstrual conditions.

Dysmenorrhea: painful menstruation with cramping

Menorrhagia: excessive menstrual bleeding lasting longer than 7 days or blood loss exceeding 80 ml (2½ ounces)

Hypomenorrhea: scanty menstrual flow (less than 1 ounce)

Metrorrhagia: irregular uterine bleeding

Polymenorrhea: episodes of menstrual bleeding occurring at less than 21-day intervals

Oligomenorrhea: menstrual cycles at greater than 35 day intervals

Folk remedies abound for painful menstruation (dysmenorrhea) and excessive menstrual bleeding (menorrhagia), but treatments for the other conditions above do not appear in most folk literature.

A common topic in folk medicine is "delayed menstruation," often discussed together with painful menstruation. Delayed menstruation refers to a brief delay of the normal period, within the normal limits above, in a woman who knows that she is not pregnant. If you experience menstrual irregularity outside the normal limits above, be sure to seek a gynecologist's advice before using folk remedies. And before treating mildly-delayed menstruation be sure that you are not pregnant.

As many as 75 percent of women have pain during menstruation at some time in their lives, and 5 to 6 percent experience incapacitating pain. The conventional treatment is pain-relieving medications, and sometimes, birth control pills to prevent ovulation. The Chinese, Ayurvedic (from India), and Arabic alternative systems of medicine believe that menstruation may be painful or slightly delayed due to a condition described as "stagnant blood." An equivalent description in modern physiology would be deficient circulation of blood to the uterus. The chief causes of stagnation, when described by traditional systems, are lack of exercise and exposure to cold weather.

The Eclectic and Physiomedicalist schools of medicine, two groups of 19th century physicians, described the same condition and treated it the same way the traditional systems did—with circulatory stimulants. Circulatory stimulants are usually hot, spicy herbs that may produce flushing of the skin and sweating, and according to traditional theories, stimulate or increase the flow of menstrual blood. These herbs are called emmenagogue herbs or foods, meaning that they stimulate the flow of the menses. These plants have not been tested in clinical trials for either pain-relieving or menstrual-promoting effects, but many of them contain antispasmodic and anti-inflammatory constituents. Use of emmenagogues is contraindicated in pregnancy, although the risk of inducing abortion with the normal amounts found in herbal teas is slight.

For any disorder of the menstrual cycle, also consider a visit to the chiropractor (D.C.) or osteopath (D.O.) to see if physical misalignment of the spine or conditions of the internal organs may be contributing to your health problem.

Remedies

GINGER: Ginger *(Zingiber officinale)* is perhaps one of the most popular—and relatively safe—menstrual cramp relievers. It is used either for delayed menstruation or for menstrual cramps in the folk medicine of the eastern United States. Ginger is used for these conditions in the folk traditions of New England, New York, and Indiana, and it is also used among the Amish in Michigan. Ginger is used for the same purposes in the traditional medical systems of China, India, and Arabia.

Ginger contains a number of anti-inflammatory constituents, including some that specifically suppress prostaglandins, which are thought to be responsible for menstrual cramping (see sidebar, "Calming Menstrual Pain," page 268). Ginger also contains four antispasmodic constituents. These actions may help menstruation to occur more naturally.

☞ DIRECTIONS: Place ½ teaspoon of ginger powder in a cup. Fill with boiling water and let stand, covered, for five minutes. Strain. Drink a cup, hot, two or three times a day, as needed.

CINNAMON: A Chinese folk remedy uses cinnamon *(Cinnamomum verum)* to stimulate delayed menses or to treat cramps. Cinnamon was used in the same way by the Eclectic physicians of the 19th and early 20th centuries. Cinnamon contains a mixture of both anti-inflammatory and antispasmodic constituents.

☞ DIRECTIONS: Place ¼ teaspoon of cinnamon powder in a cup. Fill with boiling water and let stand, covered, for five minutes. Strain. Drink a cup, hot, two or three times a day as needed.

FENNEL: Fennel seed tea *(Foeniculum vulgare)* is a treatment for menstrual cramps in Chinese folklore. Fennel, a warming spice, promotes circulation in the same manner as the other emmenagogues in this section. Fennel also contains seven different antispasmodic constituents.

☞ DIRECTIONS: Grind 1 teaspoon of fennel seeds in a coffee grinder or with a mortar and pestle. Place the fennel powder in a cup. Fill with boiling water and let stand, covered, for five minutes. Strain. Drink 1 cup of the tea, hot, three times a day.

JUNIPER BERRIES: In *American Folk Medicine,* folklorist Clarence Meyer suggests drinking a tea of juniper berries to bring on delayed menstruation. This remedy was also used in ancient Egypt, although the Egyptians made the tea with milk instead of water. (The Egyptians also used juniper berries to embalm the dead). Juniper berries contain at least nine antispasmodic constituents.

☞ DIRECTIONS: Crush 1 teaspoon of juniper berries in a coffee grinder or with a mortar and pestle. Place 1 teaspoon of the powder in a cup and fill with boiling water. Let steep for five to ten minutes, covered. Strain. Take ¼-cup doses every three or four hours. Don't take juniper if you have kidney disease, and don't take it daily for more than three weeks. Berries are aborti-facient. Avoid excessive consumption.

MOTHERWORT: The use of motherwort *(Leonurus cardiaca)* as a medicine has its roots in both American Indian and European history. The Delaware, Mohegan, Micmac, and Shinnecock tribes all used the plant as a medicine for gynecological conditions. Whether or not the plant was native to the northeastern areas of the country, where the tribes lived, is not known. The Indians may have adopted the use of the plant after it arrived with the European colonists. Because of its folk use in Britain for menstrual cramps and delayed menstruation, motherwort was a household folk medicine among British colonists in the early American colonies. It was later used in the medicine of the Eclectic and Physiomedicalist physicians during the 1800s and early 1900s.

The Europeans used motherwort as an emmenagogue and a heart medicine. In describing motherwort, the 17th century British herbalist Nicholas Culpepper wrote, "there is no better herb to drive melancholy vapours from the heart, to strengthen it and keep the mind cheerful, blithe and merry."

Motherwort is approved by the German government as a sedative for "nervous" heart symptoms, such as palpitations that accompany anxiety or stress. Chinese physicians also use the herb; they have used their native species of motherwort since at least A.D. 100 for treating menstrual disorders.

☞ DIRECTIONS: Place ½ ounce of motherwort herb (the dried flowering tops) in a 1-pint jar and cover with boiling water. Let stand twenty minutes. Strain and re-bottle. Take 1 to 2 ounces of the tea every two to four hours for up to three days. Don't take motherwort if you are also taking medication to treat a thyroid or heart condition.

BLUE COHOSH: Blue cohosh *(Caullophyllum thalactroides)* is a native North American plant widely used by American Indians in the eastern areas of the country where it grows. The Cherokee, Fox, Menimonee, Ojibwa, and Potawatomi tribes all used it either to facilitate childbirth or to treat painful or delayed menstruation. Cohosh is an Algonquin word meaning "rough with hairs"; the word was applied to several native American plants. Today we still use this original native word when referring to both blue cohosh and black cohosh *(Cimicifuga racemosa)*.

Calming Menstrual Pain

Medical researchers today think that an imbalance of prostaglandins—powerful hormonelike chemicals in the body—are responsible for menstrual pain. Prostaglandins are in all tissues, but certain varieties are concentrated in the lining of the uterus and may be responsible for the cramping of the uterine muscles. Aspirin, acetaminophen, ibuprofen, and many other pain-relieving medications inhibit prostaglandins, and this could explain why they also relieve some cases of menstrual cramps.

Many herbs traditionally used for cramps contain constituents that also inhibit prostaglandins. Ginger, perhaps the most popular emmenagogue listed here, contains four such constituents. Fennel, pennyroyal, tansy, juniper, rosemary, basil, thyme, chamomile, cinnamon, and yarrow contain such constituents as well. Although the plants themselves have not been tested for pain-relieving activity, it is possible that their constituents are responsible for some of the pain-relieving effects observed in folk medicine.

Blue cohosh was listed in the first botany books of North American plants in the 1700s and 1800s. It was introduced into medical practice in 1813 by an Indian doctor in Cincinnati named Peter Smith. From about 1850 until the early 1900s, both the Eclectic and Physiomedicalist schools of medicine considered it to be one of the most important women's medicines. The women took the plant for several weeks before childbirth to strengthen uterine contractions (it is now contraindicated for self-medication during pregnancy). Doctors also prescribed it for menstrual cramps or delayed menstruation.

Constituents in blue cohosh have been identified as uterine stimulants, or promoting contractions. Despite rumors to the contrary, blue cohosh is not a reliable abortive herb. Most likely, it will just make you feel sick.

☞ DIRECTIONS: Place ½ ounce of blue cohosh root in a pot. Cover with a pint of water. Bring to a boil and then simmer, covered, on low heat for twenty minutes. Let cool to room temperature. Strain and bottle.

GERMAN CHAMOMILE: Chamomile *(Matricaria recutita)* is considered in German medicine to be one of the most reliable herbal medicines for menstrual cramps. Chamomile is also mentioned as a cramp remedy in folk traditions throughout North America. The Latin name matricaria comes from the word "mater," meaning both mother and womb. The use of the plant for relieving cramps is probably ancient.

☞ DIRECTIONS: Place ½ ounce of chamomile in a 1-quart jar and fill with boiling water. Let stand for one hour. Strain and drink a cup every hour or two.

BASIL: Basil *(Ocimum basilicum)* is mentioned as a remedy for painful or delayed menstruation in the folk medicine of China.

continued on page 273

Aphrodisiacs and Love Potions

Few aspects of folk medicine attract more interest than traditional aphrodisiacs. Most people are familiar with the belief that oysters increase sexual desire, and many more have heard of Spanish fly. All species, including humans, are driven to reproduce, and the influence of this instinctual drive constantly permeates our thoughts and actions. The word "aphrodisiac" comes from the Greek name for the goddess of love and beauty, Aphrodite. In folk traditions, aphrodisiacs come in many different forms. There are remedies for sexual dysfunctions such as impotence and foods like oysters that serve both as a symbolic communication of amour and a hoped-for physical boost. There are also a variety of recipes that are intended either to arouse sexual desire in another (sometimes without their knowing) or to destroy someone's sexuality.

Over the centuries many foods and drugs have had a reputation for exciting sexual desire or increasing sexual capacity. Oysters are probably the best known aphrodisiac food, and their reputation seems to come from their resemblance to testicles. This illustrates the "doctrine of signatures," a very old idea that was accepted by physicians in the days when astrology and magical ideas were a part of science. According to this doctrine, medicinal substances in nature were thought to be marked by a visual indication of their proper use. This mark was their medicinal "signature." Medicines for the blood were often red, and beans were believed to be beneficial for the kidneys because of their kidneylike shape. Besides oysters, the tubers of some orchids have also been considered aphrodisiacs because their shape resembles testicles—in fact, the source of the word "orchid" is the Greek word for testicle, *orkhis*.

After oysters, onions and garlic are probably the best known "love foods" in folk tradition, but there are others. Cayenne pepper is believed to be a powerful stimulant and effective for rousing passion because it is "hot."

The very well-known aphrodisiac Spanish fly deserves mention as well. Spanish fly is a toxic substance prepared from the dried and crushed bodies of dried beetles. This preparation causes irritation of the genito-urinary tract and increases blood flow to the area. It has never been shown scientifically to produce sexual excitement, however, and it is poisonous. There have been several cases of death due to its ingestion.

Mandrake *(Mandragora officinarum)* is a medicinal plant of the nightshade family that has a dramatic sexual reputation in folk medicine. The mandrake root is often forked, giving the rough appearance of a human form with legs. Additional forks in the root sometimes look like male genitals, and these particular roots are especially prized. Mandrake growing beneath a gallows was believed to be particularly powerful. Some even believed that the mandrake grew there from the semen of hanged criminals, increasing the sexual connection. The effects of mandrake that have been identified are sedative and anesthetic, however, so it seems very unlikely that it actually is a sexual stimulant!

American ginseng *(Panax quinquefolium)* is another herb with a powerful reputation as an aphrodisiac. Ginseng root comes originally from Asian medicine traditions. It is very difficult to cultivate, so naturally occurring ginseng is very valuable. By the 19th century, the root, often called "sang" by its Appalachian gatherers, was being exported from America to Asia in large quantities. Recent investigations of ginseng credit it as an adaptogen, a sub-

Love Blood

Most magical love potions involve the use of blood. For example, from the southern United States comes the idea that if a man can secretly place some frog's blood on the woman he loves, she will be forced to fall in love with him. The most common use of blood in love potions, however, requires that a woman place a small amount of her menstrual blood in a man's food. If he consumes it, he will be powerfully attracted to her—regardless of other competitors. This use of menstrual blood is believed to bind a woman's lover or husband to her in an overpowering way—so much so that some women say their husbands will not eat their cooking during the period of menstruation! This belief continues in many communities in the United States.

stance that aids the body in adapting to stress. If there is any truth to the folk medical idea that ginseng is a sexual tonic, especially for older men, it may lie in this sort of tonic property.

Many folk aphrodisiacs seem magical, especially those love potions intended to arouse overwhelming attraction and desire in a particular person. For example, from North Carolina comes the statement that a woman can compel a man to love her by making a powder from dried leaves shaped like hearts and sprinkling it on her intended's clothing. A more dramatic recipe from North Carolina calls for moss from the skull of a murder victim that must be taken during a full moon in a cemetery. The moss is then worn around the neck as a sort of amorous amulet. Tradition also says that if you think constantly of the one you love, she will love you back!

It is also included in the folk traditions of Hispanics in the Southwest, where it is called "albacar." Basil contains unusually large quantities of the constituent caffeic acid, which has analgesic, anti-inflammatory, antispasmodic, and anti-prostaglandin activity (see "Calming Menstrual Pain," page 268). If you don't have basil on hand, you might try thyme *(Thymus vulgaris),* which also contains a high amount of caffeic acid and is included in American folk traditions.

☞ DIRECTIONS: Place 2 tablespoons of thyme or basil leaves in a 1-pint jar and fill with boiling water. Cover tightly and let cool to room temperature. Drink ½ to 1 cup each hour for painful menstruation.

RASPBERRY: The Chippewa, Cherokee, Iroquois, Kwakiutl, and Quinalt Indians have all used raspberry leaf *(Rubus spp.)* as a gynecological medicine. In contemporary folk medicine in the United States, raspberry is probably the most famous "women's" herb. No pharmacological activities have been identified to account for the beneficial effects of this herb, but the leaf is highly nutritious; it is especially rich in minerals.

For cramps, raspberry is traditionally taken throughout the month as a beverage; cumulative mineral nutrition may account for any beneficial effects on the health. One ounce of raspberry leaf contains 408 milligrams of calcium, 446 milligrams of potassium, 106 milligrams of magnesium, 3.3 milligrams of iron, and 4.0 milligrams of manganese. The manganese concentration—which is about equal to the recommended daily allowance for women—is unusually high for an

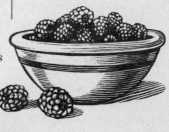

herbal source. In fact, in a sampling of 15 common herbal teas, raspberry contained about 20 times the average manganese content of the other drinks. Manganese deficiency has been associated with reproductive disorders, but not specifically with menstrual pain.

☞ DIRECTIONS: Place 1 ounce of raspberry leaf in 1 quart of water. Bring to a boil, cover, and simmer on the lowest heat for thirty to forty minutes. Let cool. Stir, strain, and bottle. Sweeten as desired. Drink the tea for two to three months.

WILLOW BARK: A New England tradition suggests taking willow bark tea *(Salix alba)* for menstrual pain. Willow bark has been used to treat arthritis, headache, and other sorts of pain in folk traditions throughout the Western world. Willow bark is approved as an analgesic by the German government. It contains salicylic acid and saligenin, compounds related to aspirin.

The "sal" in the chemical name for aspirin—acetylsalicylic acid—is named after the "sal" in the plant's genus, Salix alba.

☞ DIRECTIONS: Purchase willow bark capsules in a health food store or herb shop. Take as directed on the label. Alternatively, place 2 teaspoons of powdered willow bark in a cup, fill with boiling water, and let steep for fifteen to twenty minutes. Sweeten with honey, if desired, and drink up to four cups a day.

PENNYROYAL: Pennyroyal *(Hedeoma pulegioides),* a plant native to this country, has been used by the Cherokee and Rappahannock Indian tribes to treat menstrual pain and delayed menses. Pennyroyal (and other *Hedeoma* species) has been used by Indians as a general pain reliever. In the 1800s and early 1900s, members of the Eclectic and Physiomedicalist schools of medicine prescribed pennyroyal to treat problems associated with menstruation. Today, pennyroyal is used to treat menstrual conditions in the folk medicine of New England. In the Hispanic folk culture of the Southwest, dwarf pennyroyal *(Hedeoma nana)* is used for the same purpose.

All the above species of the plant contain salicylic acid (an aspirinlike constituent), the menstrual-promoting essential oil pulegone, and a variety of other anti-inflammatory and antispasmodic constituents. Don't ever consume the concentrated essential oil of pennyroyal, however. Pulegone is a liver toxin that caused the deaths of several women attempting to use it to induce abortion.

☞ DIRECTIONS: Place 2 tablespoons of pennyroyal herb in a 1-pint jar and fill with boiling water. Cover and let stand for one hour. Strain and take a 2-ounce dose every one to two hours. Don't take more than 1 pint a day, and don't take it for more than three days. Although it has a mintlike flavor, don't give this tea to children.

Lessening Cramps

A computer search of a U.S. Department of Agriculture database of medicinal plants for antispasmodic (cramp-relieving) activity turns up a number of traditional emmenagogue herbs. A cluster of constituents responsible for the antispasmodic activity—borneol, bornyl-acetate, limonene, and caryophyllene—appear in most of the plants included there.

Ginger, pennyroyal, tansy, juniper, rosemary, basil, thyme, cinnamon, and yarrow all have either three or four of these constituents. Chamomile has two such constituents, and fennel has one. The plants themselves have not been tested in trials for menstrual cramps and should not be used in excessive amounts.

CRAMP BARK AND BLACK HAW: Two species of the Viburnum genus, cramp bark (*Viburnum opulus*) and black haw (*Viburnum prunifolium*) have been used for treating menstrual pain and other types of spasmodic pain in American Indian medicine. (The Cherokee, Delaware, Fox, and Ojibwa tribes all used cramp bark for treating pain; the Delaware in particular used it for treating menstrual pain.) In the 1800s and early 1900s, both cramp bark and black haw were used for treating menstrual pain or delayed menses by the Eclectic and Physiomedicalist physicians.

A contemporary textbook of medical herbalism called *Lehrbuch der Phytotherapie* that's used in German medical schools recommends taking between 20 and 30 drops of cramp bark tincture or as much as one teaspoon of the tincture of either plant to treat acute menstrual cramps. Both plants contain the antispasmodic

Get Moving

In 1830, J. C. Gunn, M.D., stated that a good treatment for delayed menstruation is to keep the bowels open. Contemporary Seventh Day Adventists—members of a religious movement that advocates the use of natural remedies and alternative medicine—offer the same advice today. Physicians who practice traditional Arabic medicine and conventional German medicine follow the principle as well. Dr. Gunn also suggested moderate exercise to bring on menses, which is one of the best ways to keep bowel function healthy.

and muscle-relaxing compounds esculetin and scopoletin. Black haw also contains aspirinlike compounds.

☞ DIRECTIONS: Purchase 1 ounce each of cramp bark and black haw tincture in a health food store or herb shop. If both aren't available, either one will do. Mix them together, and take between 1 and 4 droppers every two or three hours for up to three days.

LEMON BALM: Lemon balm (*Melissa officinalis*) is used by the Amish for delayed menstruation or cramping. In the Hispanic folk tradition of the Southwest, it is used for the same purpose. The plant, which is native to southern Europe and northern Africa, now grows throughout North America as well. It has been used as a relaxing emmenagogue herb at least since the 12th century German mystic and healer Hildegarde von Bingen stated, "Lemon balm contains within it the virtues of a dozen other plants."

Lemon balm is used in traditional herbalism for a variety of conditions that arise from nervous tension. Menstruation that is delayed by stress and tension may respond best to this mild plant. Lemon balm is approved today by the German government as a sedative.

☞ DIRECTIONS: Place 1 ounce of lemon balm in a 1-quart jar and fill with boiling water. Cover tightly and let cool to room temperature. Strain and drink ½ cup per hour until the cramps are gone or your period ends.

SHEPHERD'S PURSE: Shepherd's purse (*Capsella bursa-pastoris*) is native to Europe and Asia. It became naturalized in this country in many of the areas where the early British and Spanish colonists traveled.

Shepherd's purse has been used since antiquity in Europe as a remedy for bleeding, whether from wounds or from excessive menses. The Chinese have used it to control excessive menstrual bleeding since at least A.D. 500. American Indian tribes adopted its use once it was established in North America, using it to treat severe diarrhea. Later, shepherd's purse was used for excessive menstrual bleeding by both the Eclectic and Physiomedicalist physicians in the late 19th and early 20th centuries. Shepherd's purse is named for the appearance of its seed pods, which look like small purses.

☞ DIRECTIONS: Place 1 to 2 teaspoonfuls of the dried herb in a cup and add 1 cup of boiling water. Let stand for three to five minutes. Strain and drink a cup every two to three hours just before and during the menstrual period.

YARROW: Since the time of the ancient Greeks, yarrow (*Achillea millefolium*) has been used in European traditional medicine to control bleeding, whether from war wounds or from excessive menstrual bleeding. Yarrow's scientific name, *Achillea,* comes from Achilles, one of the battlefield heroes of the Greek Iliad. Achilles reportedly used the plant to heal the wounds of his soldiers. The use of yarrow was widespread in ancient times, and names such as "military herb," "knight's millefoil," and "soldier's woundwort" survive today.

In North America, Cherokee Indian women used the plant to control heavy menstrual bleeding. Nineteenth century North American Eclectic and Physiomedicalist physicians used yarrow for treating prolonged menstrual periods. Today, yarrow is used for excessive menstrual bleeding in the folk medicine of Hispanics in the Southwest.

Besides war wounds and excessive menses, yarrow has been used by physicians of the past to reduce bleeding from hemorrhoids and intestinal ulcers. Yarrow has not been formally tested for its ability to reduce any sort of bleeding, but it contains two alkaloids—achilleine and betonicine—that have shown to reduce bleeding in animal trials.

☞ DIRECTIONS: Place ½ ounce of yarrow in a 1-pint jar and fill with boiling water. Cover and let stand until the tea reaches room temperature. For heavy menstrual bleeding, drink ½ cup every one to two hours for a day or two. Yarrow is not recommended for epileptics or during pregnancy.

Mouth, Gums, and Teeth

Dental problems are perhaps the oldest known conditions to afflict humanity. Prehistoric skulls from 25,000 years ago show signs of tooth decay. Folk remedies for tooth, mouth, and gum problems have probably existed at least since that time. By 3700 B.C., the Egyptians were using tiny drills to make a hole in the jaw to drain an infected tooth. By 2700 B.C., the Chinese had begun to treat tooth pain with acupuncture. The Greek physician Aesculapius introduced the pulling of diseased teeth in Greece sometime around 1200 B.C. It was the barbers who pulled teeth in 17th century England. Reliable dental anesthetics only became available in the United States during the 1800s; anesthetics were still not available in some isolated areas of this country as late as the early 1970s, however. Understandably, then, many folk remedies for toothache, mouth pain, and gum disease survive into present day in spite of more reliable professional dental care.

The best medicine for dental problems is prevention, which means regular cleaning of the teeth. Diet also has a strong impact on dental health, and unfortunately, our modern processed foods promote tooth decay. During the 1930s, dentist and researcher Weston Price, visited more than 20 traditional cultures, including peoples in Europe, Africa, North America, South America, Australia, and the South Sea Islands. In each place, he examined the teeth of the inhabitants who ate a traditional diet and the teeth of those who ate modern foods, which were just being introduced into their villages at that time. The people eating the traditional diets averaged from 1 to 4 percent dental cavities, while those eating the modern foods averaged from 20 to 40 percent. The culprits among the foods were sugar and white flour. Price documented his research with photographs. You can see them for yourself in his book *Nutrition and Physical Degeneration,* which is still in print today.

The chief risk of unattended dental cavities is a dental abscess—an infection at the roots of the tooth within the jaw bone. An abscess can sometimes be "silent"and cause no pain. But it may cause systemic infection and health problems far beyond the site of the infection. An abscess may require removal of the tooth. Sometimes a root canal operation is performed. In that procedure, the nerves and vascular tissue (pulp) within the tooth are removed, a disinfectant is put into the root canal, and the tooth is filled. Teeth can be "saved" in this manner and last for many decades, or even for life.

Most of the remedies in this section are for treating gum disease or sores in the mouth. If you suffer from gum disease, remember to regularly clean your teeth—you also need to floss and go for a periodic cleaning at your dentist's office. The remedies here, including the ones for dental pain, may still come in handy, though, if you are traveling in a Third

World country, camping in the wilderness, or are otherwise prevented from getting immediate dental help.

Remedies

CLOVE: Clove *(Eugenia caryophyllata)* has been used as a toothache remedy in Asia since antiquity. Later, it moved along trade routes from Europe to the Mediterranean. By 3 B.C., clove had become a universal folk remedy for dental pain in the Mediterranean. Nineteenth century dentists in both Europe and North America also used clove oil to relieve dental pain. Today, dentists use eugenol, a major ingredient in oil of clove, to relieve dental pain and to disinfect dental abscesses. Eugenol also has local anesthetic properties. Clove is still used for dental pain today in the folk medicine of New Englanders, the Amish, and Hispanics in the Southwest.

☞ DIRECTIONS: Blend up to 1 teaspoon of clove into a powder in a coffee grinder. Moisten the powder with some olive oil and pack into a cavity or area where a filling has been lost. Alternately, you can purchase clove oil at a pharmacy or health food store. Soak a cotton ball with the oil and place on the gums next to an aching tooth. Be sure to visit your dentist promptly to prevent further tooth decay.

MYRRH GUM: Myrrh gum *(Commiphora myrrha)* has been used to treat mouth problems in the Middle East and North Africa since antiquity. The use of myrrh gum later spread to India, China, and Europe along Arab trade routes. Myrrh gum, like goldenseal, is astringent and tightens up loose gums. It is also antimicrobial. (The Egyptians used it in their mummification process to prevent the bacterial degradation of the corpse.) The following toothache remedy comes from an 1846 herbal of the Thomsonian tradition.

Bad Breath

Many people use mouthwashes to treat bad breath, but, more often than not, the odor of bad breath is due to indigestion, not mouth infection. (For persistent bad breath, see the sections on "Digestion," page 162, and "Indigestion and Heartburn," page 238.)

If your bad breath is caused by a mouth infection, try any of the remedies in this section. Aromatics, such as clove, will also freshen the breath while disinfecting the mouth. In fact, in South Asia and the Middle East, it is a custom to chew on the seeds of aromatic spices such as clove, cardamom, or fennel after meals. These seeds contain antimicrobial substances as well as constituents that freshen the breath. Oftentimes, the constituents that give an herb its smell and good taste are the same ones that fight infection and reduce inflammation.

☞ DIRECTIONS: Combine 1½ ounces of myrrh gum and 1 teaspoon of cayenne pepper (*Capsicum annum*) in a jar containing a pint of brandy. Cover the jar, and shake it several times a day for a week. Strain and save the brandy. You now have a tincture. To treat a toothache, dip a cotton ball in the tincture and place it on the cavity. Be sure to see a dentist at the first opportunity to prevent further tooth decay.

To treat swollen and inflamed gums, make a mouthwash by combining a 1-ounce shot glass of the tincture with 3 ounces of water. Rinse the mouth frequently during the day.

ECHINACEA: Echinacea was a universal toothache and gum disease remedy among the American Indians of the Great Plains region. Although it formerly grew in abundance in that area, echinacea is rapidly disappearing in that region due to overharvesting for worldwide medicinal use.

Applied topically, whether to skin or gums, echinacea can promote the healing of wounds and ulcers. Constituents in *Echinacea angustifolia,* the echinacea species used by the Plains Indians, are chemically related to the constituents in prickly ash (page 287) that produce a tingling sensation and act as a local anesthetic. These constituents are not present in *Echinacea purpurea,* however, which is the species most often available in health food stores and herb shops and the one most likely to be found in your garden.

☞ DIRECTIONS: Obtain a whole or chopped *Echinacea angustifolia* root at a health food store or herb shop. Grind a small amount in a coffee grinder. Pack the powder like snuff between your cheek and the tooth next to a sore area, or pack the powder directly into a cavity. Be sure to see your dentist at the first opportunity so that tooth decay does not progress.

GOLDENSEAL AND WILLOW: The bark of various species of the willow tree (*Salix spp.*) have been used to treat mouth and gum infections by American Indian tribes throughout North America. Eskimo groups also used it to treat mouth infections. Although willow bark is famous for its aspirinlike constituents, it has antimicrobial constituents as well. The bark is also astringent, which can tone swollen gum tissues.

☞ DIRECTIONS: Place 1 ounce of willow bark in

1 quart of water. Bring to a boil, cover, and simmer on the lowest heat for twenty minutes. Remove from heat and let stand until the water reaches room temperature. Refrigerate and use as a mouthwash up to eight times a day.

GOLDENSEAL: Goldenseal (*Hydrastis canadensis*) was a famous dental remedy of the early American colonists. It was used for mouth ulcers and infected gums. The related plants goldthread (*Coptis trifolia*) and Oregon grape root (*Mahonia aquifolium, Berberis aquifolium*) were used by the American Indians for the same purpose. Like goldenseal, goldthread and Oregon grape root contain the antimicrobial constituent berberine. Of the three plants, goldenseal is probably best for treating sore and swollen gums because it also contains strong astringent constituents that may help to firm up swollen gum tissues.

☞ DIRECTIONS: In a cup, pour 1 cup of boiling water over 1 teaspoon of goldenseal root. Let steep until the water reaches room temperature. Take 1-ounce doses. Swish around the mouth thoroughly before swallowing. Do this three times a day as needed.

MYRRH GUM: A folk remedy from contemporary Kentucky for sore and swollen gums calls for equal parts of goldenseal (*Hydrastis canadensis*) and myrrh gum (*Commiphora myrrha*). The combination also appears today in the folk medicine of Utah. This remedy has its roots in

Thomsonian herbalism and Physiomedicalist medicine of the 19th century.

☞ DIRECTIONS: Purchase goldenseal tincture and myrrh gum tincture at a health food store or herb shop. Take 1 ounce of each tincture and place in an 8-ounce jar. Fill the jar with water. Cover the jar and shake well. Store the jar in the refrigerator. Use once a day as a mouthwash or up to eight times a day for active gum disease.

YERBA MANSA: What goldenseal was to the American Indians of the eastern forests (and echinacea was to the Plains Indians), yerba mansa (*Anemopsis californica*) was to the American Southwest. All three herbs were used as panaceas for a wide variety of illnesses. Spanish settlers learned the uses of yerba mansa from the Maricopa, Pima, Tewa, and Yaqui Indian tribes. ("Yerba mansa" is short for "yerba del indio manso," or "herb of the tamed Indians.") The

Eclectic school of medicine later used yerba mansa as a mucous membrane remedy.

Yerba mansa contains the volatile constituents thymol and methyl eugenol, both of which have demonstrated antimicrobial properties. Its other constituents, which are similar to those in goldenseal and myrrh gum, are astringent. Use yerba mansa for treating sores in the mouth.

☞ DIRECTIONS: Place 1 ounce of yerba mansa in 1 quart of water, bring to a boil, and simmer for twenty to thirty minutes. Let stand until cool. Refrigerate. Use as a mouthwash for gum disease or mouth sores as often as eight times a day.

PLANTAIN LEAF: Using the plantain leaf as a toothache remedy comes from the folk medicine of Mexico and of Hispanics in the American Southwest. Plantain leaf is rich in antimicrobial and antiinflammatory substances. The following recipe comes from Hispanic folk tradition in Los Angeles.

☞ DIRECTIONS: Take a small amount of lard or other oil solid. (The lard or oil should be room temperature.) "Wash" the lard first in salt water, then in vinegar water, and finally in 100 proof spirits such as vodka. Crush a plantain leaf, spread the lard on it, and then place the leaf between your cheek and sore tooth.

FIGS: A remedy from Mexico and Hispanics in the American Southwest requires cutting a fig in half and laying one half of it lengthwise between your cheek and the aching tooth. The same treatment is used in Arabic medicine. The Arab remedy calls for green figs, not ripe ones, however. The remedy may have been the result of a mixing of Spanish and Arabic customs. (The Muslims controlled Spain for 800 years, starting in the 7th century A.D.)

☞ DIRECTIONS: If you have access to a fig tree, grab a fig and cut it in half. Set one half of the fig between your cheek and tooth, with the open side facing the sore tooth.

SALT WATER: A remedy from New England for bleeding gums, canker sores, or toothache is to rinse the mouth with salt water. The same remedy is mentioned in the folklore of North Carolina. Salt, like many of the plant remedies above, is both antimicrobial and astringent, so it can shrink swollen gum tissues.

☞ DIRECTIONS: Place 1 teaspoon of salt in a cup of warm water. Rinse the mouth every two to three hours when treating an infection. North Carolina tradition suggests placing 1 teaspoon of salt directly on a sore tooth and gently biting down until the pain is relieved.

PRICKLY ASH: Prickly ash bark *(Zanthoxylum americanum)* has been used as a toothache remedy by various Indian tribes in the eastern United States; it was the most common tooth-pain remedy of the Iroquois Indians. Prickly ash is still used today in the folk medicine of the southern Appalachians and by some rural Louisiana blacks. (These two groups are sometimes beyond the reach of dental care—economically, if not geographically.) Prickly ash bark produces a tingling sensation when chewed, which soon gives way to numbness. In Louisiana, where blacks call the plant "toothache tree," the bark is crushed and then rubbed on the gums or inserted into a cavity as an anesthetic.

☞ DIRECTIONS: Prickly ash is often available in health food stores or herb shops only in tincture form. Using the tincture dropper, apply the tincture directly to the painful area. Alternately, put some of the tincture, undiluted, on a small piece of cotton and hold next to the gums.

BAKING SODA: A folk remedy from North Carolina for treating toothache pain is baking soda. The same suggestion comes from the Hispanic folk traditions of Los Angeles. Concentrated baking soda acts as a disinfectant.

☞ DIRECTIONS: Fill the hollow of the cavity in a sore tooth with baking soda. Go to the dentist as soon as possible before the decay spreads.

Muscle Strains and Sprains

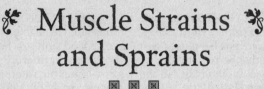

When the body's tissues are injured, the body initiates the process of inflammation to heal them. Blood flow increases to the area, causing redness. Lymph floods the tissues, causing swelling. (The initial flooding of lymph to the area can cause severe pain as the tissues are stretched.) Chemicals that cause pain are secreted to the damaged tissues. The net effect of all this swelling and pain is to immobilize the area to prevent further injury.

Next, some of the body's white blood cells migrate to the area to clear away damaged tissue. Good circulation is necessary at this stage to bring in the nutrients necessary to build new tissue and to carry away the debris of the injury.

You can decrease the pain in the area by reducing the swelling. Soak the affected part in cool water. After the first day, however, it is important to increase circulation to the injured part. To do this, treat the area with hot soaks and massage.

Folk traditions throughout North America and other parts of the world make use of irritating liniments and plasters to treat muscle injuries. These treatments are applied externally to irritate the skin at the site of the pain—a process called counterirritation. Experiments show that counterirritation not only increases blood flow to the skin by as much as four times, but also increases blood flow and temperature to the muscles underneath the injured area.

Other folk remedies for strains and sprains are taken internally and have pharmacological effects similar to aspirin.

Remedies

WINTERGREEN OIL: Wintergreen *(Gaultheria procumbens)* has been used to treat muscle pain by the Delaware, Menominee, Ojibwa, Potawatomi, and Iroquois Indian tribes. It entered into official United States medicine for this purpose in 1820 and remains, in the form of wintergreen oil, a medicine included in the *United States Pharmacopoeia.* Wintergreen and wintergreen oil also appear as treatments for muscle pain in the folk medicine of New England. The active pain-relieving constituent in wintergreen is methylsalicylate, a chemical relative of aspirin. The concentrated oil has been used as a pain-relieving medicine since the 1800s, but it can be toxic, even when applied to the skin. (Aspirin was discovered during the search for safer pain-relieving drugs.) If you want to use this plant, stick with the dried herb.

☞ DIRECTIONS: Pour 1 pint of boiling water over 1 ounce of dried wintergreen leaves in a cup. Let stand until it reaches room temperature. Apply as a wash over the affected area, and simultaneously take 2-ounce doses of the tea three to four times a day.

EPSOM SALT BATHS: Folk traditions in both New England and Indiana call for Epsom salt baths to relieve the pain of strains and sprains. The salt is composed mainly of magnesium sulfate. The heat of an Epsom salt bath can increase circulation and promote the healing of strains and sprains. The magnesium of the salt is absorbed through the skin. Magnesium is one of the most important minerals in the body, participating in at least 300 enzyme systems. It also has antiinflammatory properties. Epsom salts have been used medicinally in Europe for more than three hundred years.

☞ DIRECTIONS: Fill a bathtub with water as hot as can be tolerated. Add 2 cups of Epsom salts. Bathe for thirty minutes, adding hot water if necessary to keep the water warm.

MUSTARD PLASTER: The mustard plaster, used since the dawn of history, remains today in the folk literature of Appalachia, China, and Europe. The irritating substance in mustard is not activated until the seeds are crushed and mixed with liquid.

☞ DIRECTIONS: Crush the seeds of white mustard (*Brassica alba*) or brown mustard (*Brassica juncea*) or grind them in a seed grinder. Moisten the mixture with vinegar and sprinkle with flour. Spread the mixture on a cloth. Cover with a second cloth. Lay the moist side across the painful area. Leave on about twenty minutes. Remove if the poultice becomes uncomfortable. Wash the affected area.

CAYENNE PEPPER: In the folk medicine of Utah, Indiana, Illinois, Ohio, and China, cayenne pepper (*Capsicum spp.*) is used in liniments and plasters. Hispanics in the Southwest use cayenne pepper in their liniments as well. Cayenne became a popular folk remedy thanks to Thomsonian herbalism, which was a well-known herbal movement throughout rural New England and the Midwest in the early 1800s. A constituent of cayenne, called capsaicin, which is also used in police "pepper spray," stimulates pain receptors without actually burning the tissues. Thus, cayenne is one of the safest items to use for counterirritation.

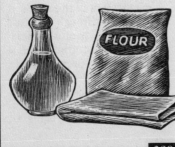

Below is a simple cayenne liniment.

☞ DIRECTIONS: Place 1 ounce of cayenne pepper in a quart of rubbing alcohol. Let the solution stand for two to three weeks, shaking the bottle each day. (You'll need to make this one in advance!) Then apply to the affected area. (This remedy is not for internal use.)

A faster alternative is to place 1 ounce of cayenne pepper in 1 pint of boiling water. Simmer for half an hour. Do not strain, but add 1 pint of rubbing alcohol. Let cool to room temperature. Apply as desired.

Probably the fastest method, from contemporary North American Chinese folklore, is to gently melt 5 teaspoons of petroleum jelly in a pan and add to it 1 teaspoon of cayenne pepper. Stir well and allow to cool to room temperature. Apply as desired.

ROSEMARY: Rosemary (*Rosmarinus officinalis*) was used to relieve pain and spasm by doctors of the Physiomedicalist school in the last century. Today, rosemary is used (both externally and internally) in the folk medicine of Mexico and the Southwest for treating the pain of pulled muscles. Rosemary contains four anti-inflammatory substances, including rosmarinic acid, which has a biochemical action similar to aspirin. Rosmarinic acid is also easily absorbed through the skin and is approved as a topical analgesic by the German government.

☞ DIRECTIONS: Put 1 ounce of rosemary leaves in a 1-pint canning jar and fill with boiling water. Cover tightly and let stand for thirty minutes. Apply as a wash over the painful area two to three times a day. Each time you apply the wash, drink a 2-ounce dose of the wash as well.

WITCH HAZEL: Witch hazel is a tree native to North America. It contains both astringent and anti-inflammatory properties. Settlers learned the use of witch hazel for treating

Chinese "Hit" Medicine

One branch of traditional Chinese herbal medicine, called "hit medicine", deals with the treatment of traumatic injuries. In any North American Asian market that sells herbal remedies, you can find these internal and external medicines for strains, sprains, and bruises. Liniments and plasters that stick to your skin and other formulas are all available. Some formulas to look for are Yunnan Pi Yao, an internal formula shown in clinical trials to reduce internal bleeding and bruising; White Flower Analgesic Balm, an external liniment; and Po Sum On medicated oil, which is also for external use.

pain from the Indians of the Oneida tribe in New York. In the 1840s, the use of the plant spread throughout the United States in the form of various over-the-counter products. The use of witch hazel later spread to Europe, where its extract became popular. Witch hazel extract remains in use today in professional British herbalism and in conventional German medicine. The German government has approved the use of witch hazel for treating minor inflammations, especially of the skin and mucous membranes.

Witch hazel is also used in the folk medicine of New England as an external application for sprains.

☞ DIRECTIONS: Purchase a witch hazel liniment at your pharmacy. Apply the liniment externally over the painful area three to four times a day. Do this as often as desired.

ARNICA: Arnica has long been used in European folk medicine to treat injuries. The use of arnica entered into regular medical practice by the time of the colonization of North America; European physicians and folk healers brought the knowledge with them. Some American Indian groups used arnica for strains and sprains—much like the Europeans did. The herb is indigenous to Europe and Siberia, but it has been naturalized in southwestern Canada and the western United States. Do not use arnica ointments and liniments on broken skin, however. Arnica acts as a counterirritant and can sometimes irritate the skin.

☞ DIRECTIONS: Pick arnica flowers (if they grow in your area) and place them in a jar. Cover the flowers with rubbing alcohol and allow to soak for two to three weeks. Shake the jar daily. Then use as a liniment for sore muscles, bruises, and backaches.

Alternately, you can try this Gypsy remedy: Purchase an arnica tincture. Use 2 tablespoons of tincture per pint of water. Apply the diluted tincture with a piece of gauze to the affected area. Tape the gauze in place. Reapply every half hour. (Note: Arnica is poisonous. It is not for internal use. Keep out of reach of children.)

❧ Nausea and Vomiting ❧

Nausea is an extremely uncomfortable or queasy feeling in the stomach area, often accompanied by an urge to vomit. Vomiting is the forceful ejection of the contents of the stomach through the mouth.

The sensation of nausea and the urge to vomit originate in an area of the brain called the vomiting center. In response to certain messages from nerves in the digestive system or in the inner ear (part of which controls balance) or to direct stimulation by certain drugs, the vomiting center can trigger the muscular actions that result in vomiting.

Nausea most often follows food poisoning or bacterial or viral infections of the intestinal tract. The nausea center can also be stimulated by ear infections, head trauma, or other neurological conditions in the brain such as migraine headache. Poisons in the bloodstream, such as alcohol, can also trigger nausea and induce vomiting. Severe vomiting, vomiting with pain as a predominant symptom, vomiting after a head injury, or chronic nausea all require medical diagnosis and treatment. Other common causes of nausea or vomiting are prescription drugs and pregnancy.

Nausea and vomiting are usually temporary conditions that can be beneficial if they result in the expulsion of something potentially harmful to the body. However, persistent or recurring vomiting can lead to a dangerous loss of fluids and salts (called dehydration) and nutrients. This risk of dehydration is most serious in infants and the elderly, but it is also a threat in individuals with bulimia, a condition in which vomiting is induced in order to control weight gain.

Conventional treatment for simple nausea is to drink clear fluids and, if vomiting has subsided, eat dry or bland foods such as soda crackers. Pediatric electrolyte replacement fluids, available in most supermarkets and pharmacies, may be the best treatment for children and the elderly. Conventional physicians can also prescribe a variety of drugs that can successfully control the urge to vomit.

Herbal folk remedies may work in several ways. Most

of the herbs are aromatic and contain volatile oils with anti-inflammatory, antispasmodic, anesthetic, and antimicrobial properties. Their ability to relieve nausea is due to the herbs' gastrointestinal local "anesthetic" effect, according to R.F. Weiss, M.D., author of *Lehrbuch der Phytotherapie* (translation: *Herbal Medicine),* the standard textbook of medical herbalism used in German schools of medicine and pharmacy. When ingested, says Weiss, the herbs work by numbing the nerve endings of the stomach, thereby reducing the gag reflex.

Remedies

MINT: Mints such as peppermint *(Mentha piperita)* and spearmint *(Mentha spicata)* are used throughout North America and Europe for soothing nausea. The Cherokee, Micmac, and Cheyenne Indians all used mints for this purpose. Today, mints are recommended for nausea in the folk tradi-

tions of Indiana and in the Hispanic folklore of the Southwest. Mints are also used to soothe nausea in contemporary Arabic medicine.

Peppermint was used medicinally by the ancient Egyptians and was also valued by the Greeks and Romans. The 17th century British herbalist Nicholas Culpepper wrote that "few remedies are of greater efficacy" for nausea than peppermint. Peppermint is approved in Germany as a medicine for weak digestion, and, according to a German textbook on medical herbalism, nausea is one of the top indications for using peppermint. The plant may reduce the gag reflex by anesthetizing the stomach lining.

☞ DIRECTIONS: Place 1 tablespoon of mint leaves in a 1-pint jar and fill with boiling water. Let stand twenty to thirty minutes, shaking the bottle from time to time to mix its contents. Strain and sip as desired.

continued on page 298

Preventing Morning Sickness

❖ ❖ ❖

The nausea and vomiting of early pregnancy, usually referred to as "morning sickness," are two of the most notable pregnancy symptoms. (This condition was written about as early as 2000 B.C.) The term morning sickness is actually a misnomer because the symptoms can happen at any time of day. The severity and occurrence of morning sickness vary not only from woman to woman, but also from pregnancy to pregnancy in the same individual.

According to present day medical opinion, the cause of morning sickness is still unclear. Some findings, however, do suggest that increased production of the HCG (human chorionic gonadotropin) hormone is a contributing factor and slowed digestion, anxiety, and emotional stress can make the problem worse. Today's physicians and midwives recommend eating a carbohydrate, such as crackers or a banana, before rising to prevent nausea and eating small amounts of nongreasy foods throughout the day. Other specialists also recommend taking a B6 vitamin supplement daily or eating natural sources of B6, such as brewer's yeast and yogurt. Eating ginger, an ancient herbal treatment for nausea, is now also recognized by modern medicine as being helpful.

Although nausea is a problem for most women only during the first trimester, it is so common that folk remedies and explanations abound. Herbal and food remedies to prevent morning sickness are very common. One folk remedy recommends eating two soda crackers before getting up in the morning—exactly the remedy prescribed by today's health specialists! The Cherokee Indians used gold-enseal *(Hydrastis canadensis),* which grows wild in the woods of eastern North America, for morning sickness. A preventive from Indiana is to drink one teaspoonful of apple cider vinegar mixed in a glass of water. One from Utah recommends eating a chocolate candy bar before getting out of bed. Another Utah remedy is to eat raw eggs, a recommendation that many queasy pregnant women might find hard to follow! More advice from Utah is that the pregnant woman should just accept morning sickness because it is actually an indication that the infant will be healthier and the delivery easier. Some medical evidence does in fact indicate that those women who experience nausea in early pregnancy are less likely to have miscarriages.

Folk belief also suggests that morning sickness can indicate the sex of the baby. In Utah, if morning sickness is pronounced, then you are sure to have a girl. In other parts of the country, it is believed the opposite will result. Another belief in Utah ascribes the color of the pills taken for nausea during pregnancy to be the determining factor in the sex of the child. It is believed that blue pills will bring a boy and pink pills, a girl. In Utah, it is also believed that the baby's sex can be predicted by the physical symptoms that the father feels (called the couvade syndrome). If, instead of the mother, the expectant father feels nauseous, it is believed the baby will be a boy.

YARROW: Yarrow (*Achillea spp.*) has been used as an antiemetic by American Indians of the Iroquois, Cheyenne, and Shoshone tribes. It is used for the same purpose in European folk tradition. Yarrow contains anti-inflammatory and anesthetic constituents. These constituents probably account for any effectiveness that the herb has for treating nausea.

☞ DIRECTIONS: Place 1 tablespoon of dried yarrow leaves in a 1-pint jar and fill with boiling water. Cover and let stand for twenty to thirty minutes, turning or shaking the bottle from time to time. Strain and take sips of the warm tea. Don't take yarrow during pregnancy.

Herbs and Pregnancy

Some traditions suggest drinking coffee or black or green tea for nausea. However, all caffeine-containing drinks should be avoided during pregnancy. And, although it is still a matter of scientific debate, some trials show increased risk of miscarriage and lower birth weight for babies of mothers who consume as little as a single cup of coffee a day.

Many of the herbs in this section are contraindicated in pregnancy, especially during early pregnancy when morning sickness is most common. However, mint, ginger (doses less than 5 grams per day), chamomile, raspberry, and fennel are safe for use in the dosages recommended here, according to standard texts on botanical safety. The use of herbs such as catnip, cinnamon, clove, ginger (doses greater than 5 grams per day), thyme, and yarrow, especially in medicinal doses, should be avoided during pregnancy. Normal amounts of cinnamon, ginger, or thyme that are present in spiced foods probably present no problem, however.

GINGER: Ginger (*Zingiber officinale*) is used for treating nausea in the folk traditions of New England and China. It is also approved for treating nausea by the German government. Scientific trials have shown that ginger may reduce nausea caused by several conditions, including motion sickness, morning sickness, and the nausea that accompanies chemotherapy. Doses as low as one gram have shown this effect. Ginger contains a variety of anti-inflammatory and local gastrointestinal anesthetic constituents.

☞ DIRECTIONS: Place ½ teaspoon of powdered ginger spice in a cup. Fill with boiling water. Cover and let stand for ten minutes. Strain the tea and drink in sips. Don't drink more than three cups of ginger tea per day during pregnancy. And don't drink ginger tea without consulting your doctor if you have gallstones.

RASPBERRY LEAF TEA: The Amish suggest a tea of raspberry leaves (*Rubus idaeus*) for treating nausea. The Thompson and Kwakiutl Indians used the leaves of related members of the Rubus genus in the same manner. No specific antinauseant or anesthetic properties have been identified in raspberry leaf constituents, but the tannin constit-uents in the leaves may have an anti-inflammatory or soothing effect on the digestive tract wall.

☞ DIRECTIONS: Place 1 ounce of raspberry leaves in a 1-quart jar. Fill with boiling water. Cover and let the tea stand until it reaches room temperature. Shake the bottle from time to time to mix its contents. Drink raspberry leaf tea as often as you wish.

GERMAN CHAMOMILE: Chamomile tea (*Matricaria recutita*) has been used as a nausea remedy by the Cherokee Indians. It continues to be used in the folk traditions of New England. Chamomile contains powerful anti-inflammatory and analgesic substances that may reduce the gag reflex. Chamomile is approved as a digestive remedy by the German government, although not specifically for nausea.

☞ DIRECTIONS: Place 2 tablespoons of chamomile flowers in a 1-pint jar and fill with boiling water. Let stand twenty to thirty minutes, shaking the bottle from time to time to mix its contents. Strain and sip as desired.

CHAMOMILE AND MINT: An antinausea formula found in the folk traditions of the Kentucky Appalachian mountains is a combination of chamomile and peppermint. The two herbs are more often used together than separately.

☞ DIRECTIONS: Place 1 tablespoon each of chamomile flowers and peppermint leaves in a 1-pint jar and fill with boiling water. Let stand twenty to thirty minutes, shaking the bottle from time to time to mix its contents. Strain and sip as desired.

CINNAMON: A nausea remedy from the folk traditions of Hispanics in the Southwest, and also from China, is cinnamon *(Cinnamomum verum)*. Called "canela" in the Southwest, cinnamon contains anti-inflammatory, anesthetic, and pain-relieving constituents. Cinnamon is approved as a digestive aid in Germany, although not specifically for nausea.

☞ DIRECTIONS: Place ½ teaspoon of cinnamon powder in a cup, and fill with boiling water. Cover and let steep for five minutes. Strain and drink sips of the tea as desired for nausea. Don't take cinnamon during pregnancy— other than in the small amounts used to season foods.

FENNEL SEED: Fennel seed *(Foeniculum vulgare)* is a nausea remedy from the folk medicine of China. It is used in traditional medicine throughout Chinatowns in North America, usually in combination with other plants.

Electrolyte Replacement Therapy

The main health hazard of excessive vomiting is dehydration and the loss of electrolyte salts. Replacement drinks are available in supermarkets and pharmacies, or you can make your own. The World Health Organization formula for an electrolyte replacement beverage after excessive diarrhea or vomiting is:

   3.5 grams sodium chloride (table salt)
   2.5 grams sodium bicarbonate (baking soda)
   1.5 grams potassium chloride (must be obtained from a pharmacy)
   20 grams of glucose (also available from a pharmacy)
   1 liter of water (1 quart and 2 ounces)

A German medical text suggests the following formula, which includes peppermint (*Mentha piperita*) and fennel (*Foeniculum vulgare*), two folk herbs often used in treating nausea: Make a tea by simmering 1 tablespoon each of peppermint leaves and fennel seed in 1 quart of water for 15 minutes in a covered pot. Strain and allow to cool to room temperature. To this add $^1/_2$ teaspoon salt, $^1/_4$ teaspoon of baking soda, $^1/_4$ teaspoon potassium chloride, and 2 tablespoons of glucose. Drink freely.

Fennel contains anesthetic constituents that may reduce the stomach's gag reflex. Also, its constituent anethole has antiseptic and antispasmodic properties.
   ☞ DIRECTIONS: Crush 1 tablespoon of fennel seeds in a coffee grinder. Place the crushed seeds in a cup and fill with boiling water. Cover and let steep for ten minutes. Drink the tea in sips for nausea.
   continued on page 304

In Hopes of Fertility

❖ ❖ ❖

Folk traditions for fertility fall into two categories. There are customs that are designed to insure fertility and there are practices to deal with the problem of infertility.

Many hopeful symbols of growth and abundance cluster around the marriage ceremony and the early days of a marriage. Throwing rice, corn, or wheat at the wedding, for instance, represents the guests' wishes for a fertile union. It is good luck to include small children in the wedding party; the presence of infants and children is representative of "sympathetic" magic (like attracting like).

A three-part custom says that the couple should eat rice at the wedding for fertility, drink wine for the pleasures of life, and sip vinegar so they will share all of life's bitterness and trouble together. A variation of that custom is for the couple to bring salt, bread, and wine into their new house to insure that they will be fertile and never lack for food or drink. Also to promote fertility, besides being carried by the groom, the bride can carry a baby over the threshold. The couple can also have their mothers make the bed, or they can put a leafy branch or a baby on it.

If all these practices failed and the couple was not soon expecting, there were a number of things they could do. The couple could maximize their chances of getting pregnant by making love during a full moon. Also, there were several patent medicines of the past that promised "a baby in every bottle." Or, a sister of the would-be mother could lay her baby on their bed. (It was even luckier if the baby urinated there.) The couple could try putting salt in their bed or garlic under the pillow. Or they could eat the garlic, which is believed to be second only to eggs in promoting fertility. Other recommended foods include oysters (a well-known aphrodisiac), olives, onions, fish, mistletoe juice, cornflower tea, and mandrake root. The couple also could turn to magic or religion, such as tying a red ribbon around the finger of a deceased relative to remind him to intercede on their behalf when he appeared before God. One elaborate ritual suggested that the couple learn alternating verses of the story of Genesis in the Bible and repeat them to one other, a verse at a time, on alternate days, just before intercourse. A very common magical belief was that if a childless couple adopted a child, biological children would follow.

This lore demonstrates the well-known anthropological theory that people resort to magical thinking when events seem beyond their control. It also reveals the deep emotional investment in the idea of children.

Sometimes, of course, it wasn't fertility that was the problem. It was that offspring could grow too numerous. "A poor man will always have many children," goes one saying, which was used to console him for his poverty (or perhaps explain it!). Folk methods of contraception did not seem to offer much for the overburdened pair, since it is often at odds with biological science: cola or vinegar douches, and coitus while standing, sitting, or with the woman on top. Some women still believe that they are more likely to get pregnant during their period than the rest of the month. This is because they envision their wombs as "open" to let out menstrual flow and "closed" the rest of the month. Of course, the exact opposite, timing-wise, is true.

A pregnant woman can become a source of further fecundity. Perfect strangers may ask to touch her stomach for luck. And, whereas menstruating women, being temporarily "sterile," were supposed to avoid tasks like planting or baking, a pregnant woman might be asked to lend her hand to these types of endeavors where increase was desired.

POPCORN: A nausea remedy from Indiana folk medicine calls for eating popcorn. The popcorn should be popped without oil, and then covered with boiling water. The result: a bland mush. The recommendation is consistent with the orthodox medical advice to eat bland food such as soda crackers for nausea.

☞ DIRECTIONS: Pop the popcorn in a skillet with a lid, without using oil. Place the dry popcorn in a bowl. Cover with boiling water and let stand for fifteen minutes. Eat a teaspoon of the soggy popcorn every ten minutes.

CLOVE: Clove (*Syzygium aromaticum*) is used for nausea in the Hispanic folk traditions of the Southwest. The spice is also used throughout Southeast Asia, South Asia, the Middle East, North Africa, and Spain for the same purpose. Clove is one of the most important herbal remedies for treating nausea in traditional Indian and Arabic medicine as well. Eugenol, the main constituent of the aromatic clove oil, is used by dentists for its powerful antiseptic and anesthetic properties.

☞ DIRECTIONS: Place 1 teaspoon of clove powder in a cup and fill with boiling water. Cover and let steep for five minutes. Strain and drink sips of the tea as desired for nausea. Don't use clove during pregnancy—other than in the small amounts used to season foods.

CATNIP: Catnip, a nausea remedy and sedative in European folk traditions, came to North America with the European colonists and quickly became naturalized here. The Iroquois Indians adopted its use both as a sedative, especially for children, and a digestive remedy. Catnip contains aromatic anti-inflammatory and anesthetic constituents.

☞ DIRECTIONS: Place 2 tablespoons of catnip leaves in a 1-pint jar and fill with boiling water. Cover and allow to stand for twenty to thirty minutes. Strain and drink by the sip for nausea. Don't use catnip as a medicine during pregnancy.

❧ Pain ❧

▨ ▨ ▨

Pain is an unpleasant or uncomfortable sensation that can range from mild irritation to excruciating agony. It is probably the most commonly reported symptom and is linked to innumerable disorders and diseases.

Pain occurs when specialized nerve endings are stimulated; within a fraction of a second this pain "signal" travels through a network of nerves to the brain. Pain can be a warning sign, indicating impending damage to the body, or it can be a protective mechanism, causing the person feeling pain to remove the cause or reflexively draw away from the source.

Most healthy people have occasional, brief twinges of pain that have no specific cause and are usually harmless. However, bothersome, recurring, or persistent pain can be caused by thousands of factors. Most commonly, pain is a symptom of disease, injury, or abnormal changes in the body.

There are many types of pain. Pain can be dull and constant, sharp and sudden, crushing, burning, piercing, or aching. When it is felt in areas other than the location of the disorder (for example, when the pain of heart attack is felt in the arm), it is called referred pain. Unexplainable pain should be reported promptly to a doctor for investigation and possible treatment.

Using plants to quiet pain goes back before the dawn of recorded medical history, but none of these plants proved particularly effective. That is why this century brought about newer and better pain drugs and why pain medications are among the most popular over-the-counter drugs. Many of the modern drugs, such as aspirin, acetaminophen, ibuprofen, and corticosteroids, suppress the formation of prostaglandins, a class of chemicals in the local tissues that trigger pain. There are other, more potent painkillers, such as the opiates morphine and codeine, but these must be prescribed by a doctor.

Many of the plants used in folk medicine for pain relief use the same biochemical pathways as the non-opiate pain-relieving drugs, but they are not as effective. On the other hand, many of these plants have multiple effects. Their antispasmodic and circulation-promoting constituents may make up for what these plants lack in prostaglandin-suppressing strength. Comparative trials of these plants with drugs have not been performed, but the plants' persistent use in folk medicine (even with the availability of inexpensive over-the-counter drugs) indicates that they must have at least some beneficial effect. Herbal formulas that combine prostaglandin-suppressing, antispasmodic, sedative, and antidepressant plants are commonly prescribed by professional herbalists in North America, Great Britain, and Australia (see sidebar, "Formulas for Chronic Pain," right).

Folk traditions throughout North America and other parts of the world also make use of irritating liniments and plasters to treat muscle and joint pain. These remedies are applied externally to irritate the skin over the site of the pain. Physiological tests show that such treatments increase blood flow to the skin by as much as four times and also increase blood flow and temperature in the muscles underneath the skin. Any relief from such treatments is due to this increased circulation to the area, which ensures a healthy flow of oxygen to the tissues and relieves the swelling of stagnant lymph in the area. This method, called counterirritation, may also increase local or systemic levels of endorphins, the body's natural pain-killing substances that are more potent than opiates.

Remedies

HOT PEPPERS: Cayenne pepper *(Capsicum spp.)* is used in formulas for

Formulas for Chronic Pain

Although acute pain may be best treated with pharmaceutical drugs, medical herbalists of countries such as Great Britain, North America, Australia, and New Zealand often use combinations of herbs and hydrotherapy to treat chronic pain. Chronic pain often creates a constellation of problems—besides the pain itself, tension, spasm, insomnia, or depression can often result. And while conventional pain medications may remedy one or two of these side effects, some formulas of herbs can address them all. A pain-reliever, an antispasmodic, a sedative, and an antidepressant may all be in included in a typical herbal formula created by a medical herbalist. For example, one herbal combination may include equal parts of willow bark (for pain), cramp bark (for spasm), valerian (a sedative), and St. John's wort (an antidepressant).

liniments and plasters in the folk medicine of China, the American Southwest, Utah, and throughout Ohio, Indiana, and Illinois. External and internal use of cayenne pepper to stimulate circulation was a key element of Thomsonian herbalism throughout rural New England and the Midwest in the early 1800s. (The Thomsonian movement of folk herbalism was introduced into practice in the early 19th century by Samuel Thomson, an influential New England herbalist. Thomsonian herbalism has been a powerful influence on American folk herbal traditions for the last 190 years.) Capsaicin, a constituent of cayenne, stimulates pain receptors without actually burning the tissues. Cayenne is thus one of the safest items to use for counterirritation. Below is a simple cayenne liniment.

☞ DIRECTIONS: Place 1 ounce of cayenne pepper in a quart of rubbing alcohol. Let the mixture stand for three weeks, shaking the bottle each day. Then, apply to the affected part during acute attacks.

Alternately, if you can't wait three weeks for relief, try this method: Place 1 ounce of cayenne pepper in a pint of boiling water. Simmer for half an hour. Do not strain, but add a pint of rubbing alcohol. Let cool to room temperature. Apply as desired to the affected part. (Do not ingest either of these remedies.)

CRAMP BARK AND BLACK HAW: For the treatment of spasmodic pain, both cramp bark (*Viburnum opulus*) and black haw (*Viburnum prunifolium*) have been used in American Indian medicine. The Cherokee, Delaware, Fox, and Ojibwa tribes all used cramp bark to treat both menstrual pain and muscle spasm. Cramp bark and black haw were used for arthritic or menstrual pain in Physiomedicalist and Eclectic medicine. The plants contain the antispasmodic

Compresses, Poultices, and Liniments

You can use compresses to treat headache, sore muscles, itching, and swollen glands, among other conditions. To make a compress, soak a cloth in a strong herbal tea, wring it out, and place it on the skin.

To make a poultice or plaster, mash herbs with enough water to form a paste. Place the herb mash directly on the affected body part and cover with a clean white cloth or gauze.

A liniment is a topical preparation that contains alcohol or oil and stimulating warming herbs such as cayenne. Sometimes isopropyl, or rubbing, alcohol is used instead of grain alcohol. Do not take products made with rubbing alcohol internally. Historically, liniments have been the treatment of choice for aching rheumatic joints and chronic lung congestion.

and muscle-relaxing compounds esculetin and scopoletin. The antispasmodic constituents are best extracted with alcohol (rather than water), so tinctures may be more effective than teas. Black haw also contains aspirin-like compounds.

☞ DIRECTIONS: Purchase 1 ounce each of cramp bark and black haw tincture in a health food store or herb shop. If both aren't available, either one will do. Mix them together, and take between 1 and 4 droppers every two or three hours for up to three days.

GINGER: Ginger is used to treat various sorts of pain in the folk medicine of China. It is also used for pain or spasm in the folk medicine of New England, Appalachia, North Carolina, and Indiana. It is an important pain medication in contemporary Arabic medicine; reports of its use there in treating migraine headache and arthritis

Homeopathic Remedies

Homeopathic medicine is based on the principle of similars, the idea that "like cures like." Homeopathic medicine holds that a substance that causes certain symptoms when given in large doses to a healthy person can cure an ill person with the same symptoms when given in very small doses. This idea that the same substance that can cause symptoms can also be used to heal is often met with skepticism.

Homeopathic remedies are highly diluted substances and are thus a subject of controversy in science. In fact, some are so diluted that they contain no traces of the original substance. Although clinical trials have shown that some homeopathic remedies do have a medicinal effect, conventional scientists have yet to prove how they work.

Perhaps the most popular homeopathic remedy sold in United States health food stores for treating pain is arnica, though it has not withstood the validity tests of clinical trials. Undiluted arnica contains various anti-inflammatory and wound-healing substances and has been used as a pain medication in the past. Users of homeopathic arnica claim the herb relieves traumatic pain that is accompanied by bruising. However, at least five clinical trials have shown that it works no better than a placebo. It was tested for the pain accompanying abdominal surgery, tooth extraction, and heavy exercise. Tests of homeopathic arnica for surgical or dental trauma have also shown the herb to be no better than a placebo for treating pain from those conditions.

show its effectiveness. Ginger contains 12 different aromatic anti-inflammatory compounds, including some with mild aspirin-like effects.

☞ DIRECTIONS: Cut a fresh ginger root (about

the size of your thumb) into thin slices. Place the slices in a quart of water. Bring to a boil, and then simmer on the lowest possible heat for thirty minutes in a covered pot. Let cool for thirty more minutes. Strain and drink ½ to 1 cup, sweetened with honey, as desired.

WILLOW BARK: Willow bark *(Salix alba)* was used for treating pain by the ancient Greeks more than 2,400 years ago. American Indians throughout North America, from the Houma in Louisiana and Alabama to the Ninivak Eskimos in the Arctic, used it as a pain reliever even before the arrival of the European colonists. Investigation of salicin, a pain-relieving constituent in willow bark, led to the discovery of aspirin in 1899. Although aspirin is now the top-selling pain-relieving drug in the world, willow bark is still used for treating pain in the folk medicine of Indiana, New England, and the Southwest, as well as by professional medical herbalists throughout the English-speaking world. The German government has approved the use of willow bark by conventional physicians for pain and fever. The most important active constituent is salicin, but other anti-inflammatory constituents also appear in the willow bark.

☞ DIRECTIONS: Purchase willow bark capsules in a health food store or herb shop. Take as directed on the label. Also, you can place 2 teaspoons of powdered willow bark in a cup, fill with boiling water, and let steep for fifteen to twenty minutes. Sweeten with honey if desired, and drink up to four cups a day for five to seven days.

ROSEMARY: Drinking rosemary tea for pain is a

continued on page 315

Curanderismo

Curanderismo is the Spanish name for a folk healing system found primarily among Mexican Americans and Mexican nationals. The healers are called curanderos (curanderas if the healers are female), which simply means "curer." Although other Spanish-speaking populations also have folk healers called curanderos, and many of the beliefs and practices are very similar, the name curanderismo is particularly applied to the folk-healing system of Mexico. This system bears the influences of the beliefs, healing practices, and medicinal plants of both the New World and its native peoples, and of the Spaniards who conquered and governed Mexico in the 16th and 17th centuries.

Curanderismo blends material and magical as well as natural and supernatural elements in its approaches to prevention and healing. A person's health is considered to include physical, mental, emotional, and spiritual aspects and all of these aspects are believed to interact. For example, a physical sickness can be brought on by emotional or spiritual causes; an emotional illness or spiritual crisis can be brought on by physical illness. And, as might be expected, the act of healing also focuses on these aspects. In fact, healing is usually approached through two or more of these avenues, despite what the diagnosis is.

While the system of curanderismo focuses on all of these aspects, most curanderos work primarily on what they call "the material level." The healers use herbs, massage, and other physical treatments. They also use some form of prayer as well as several other approaches that may not seem "material" to those outside curanderismo. A smaller number of healers may specialize in spiritual or "mental level" diagnosis and treatments, similar to psychic healing efforts. The skills of these spiritual specialists are often sought by family members of someone who has been ill for a very long time, who has a terminal disease, or whose health problems seem to be mainly mental, spiritual, emotional, or behavioral in nature. Curanderos often refer patients to regular medical doctors in addition to offering treatments themselves.

When people go to a curandero, they usually have already tried some form of first aid and self-care and have not been satisfied with the results. People go to these respected community healers to be treated for every kind of sickness, from common childhood complaints such as colic, thrush, and measles to cancer and tuberculosis, as

Scared to Death

Susto, which means "fright," is one of the best known of the Latino folk illnesses, and it is specifically treated by curanderos. It is caused by severe fright or emotional shock—such as the startle one gets when witnessing an accident or receiving unexpected bad news. It is believed that this shock may cause a person's soul to be separated from their body. If the soul cannot return, the person will begin to feel depressed and disinterested in life, he will lose sleep and his appetite, and he will become anxious at small things.

The friends and family members of an individual who has susto should bring him to a curandero promptly, because susto is a serious condition. Studies done in Mexico confirm that people with susto recover better when they are treated by a curandero than when they are treated by a psychiatrist.

well as specific folk illnesses. People may also seek the services of a curandero when they have reason to believe that the cause of their troubles is magical or supernatural in origin. In this tradition, it is believed possible to be made sick by such influences as the evil eye or hexes.

The curandero will listen to the patient's description of the problem (and the descriptions given by their accompanying family members), ask probing questions, and try to understand the history of the presenting illness. The healer will then make his or her own diagnosis. In addition to looking, listening, and questioning, diagnosis can involve the healer's intuition, help from guiding spirits, and sometimes a form of divination, such as breaking an egg into a glass of tap water or holy water, passing the glass over the patient and interpreting the behavior of the egg in the water (sinking, rising, yolk separating from whites, etc.) to understand the nature of the problem. Spirits and divinations, if they are used, typically apply to cases in which there seems to be an important spiritual aspect to the sickness.

Once the diagnosis is made or confirmed, the curandero will usually give some treatment, as well as prescribe treatments and actions to be followed by the patient later. Treatments may include administration of herbal teas, wrapping the patient in blankets to "sweat out the illness," prayers, counseling, and "sweeping" of the body with specific herbs, raw eggs, or other objects. The principle at work in the sweepings is that of transference: It is the idea that disease, impurities, or evil elements may be transferred out of the body of the patient and into the sweeping substance, which can later be safely discarded. Particularly when the disease is strong or the causes are spiritual or supernatural, eggs may be used for sweepings. Because eggs contain the cells of life, sickness and other bad elements may transfer into these potential living forms instead of remaining with the patient.

remedy used in the contemporary Hispanic folk medicine of Mexico and the Southwest. Rosemary has not been tested in clinical trials, but it was used to relieve pain and spasm by doctors of the Physiomedicalist school in the last century. Its leaf also contains four anti-inflammatory substances—carnosol, oleanolic acid, rosmarinic acid, and ursolic acid. Carnosol acts on the same anti-inflammatory pathways as both steroids and aspirin; rosmarinic acid acts through at least two separate anti-inflammatory biochemical pathways; and ursolic acid, which makes up about 4 percent of the plant by weight, has been shown in animal trials to have anti-arthritic effects.

☞ DIRECTIONS: Put ½ ounce of rosemary leaves in a 1-quart canning jar and fill the jar with boiling water. Cover tightly and let stand for thirty minutes. Drink a cup as hot as possible before going to bed, and have another cupful in the morning before breakfast.

Hydrotherapy for Pain

During the 19th century in the United States, hydrotherapy was a popular form of medical treatment, especially for pain. The practice survives today mainly in the Appalachians and among the Seventh Day Adventists. (Hydrotherapy is also taught in naturopathic medical schools.)

Cold water or ice is recommended for acute pain; the cold suppresses inflammation and swelling. Hot water or alternating hot and cold water (ending with cold) is the prescription for chronic pain. Hot water or alternating hot and cold water increases local circulation and has the same benefits as counterirritation. Also, research shows that full body immersion (up to the neck) reduces swelling in inflamed joints.

EPSOM SALT BATHS: Folk traditions in both New England and Indiana call for Epsom salt baths to relieve pain. Epsom salt was named after a salt found in abundance in spring water near the town of Epsom, England, in 1618. The salt was reputed to have magical healing properties. Epsom salt is now produced industrially and not from the springs in England. Epsom salt is primarily magnesium sulfate and has been used medicinally in Europe for more than three hundred years. The heat of an Epsom salt bath can increase circulation and reduce the swelling of arthritis, and the magnesium can be absorbed through the skin. Magnesium is one of the most important minerals in the body, participating in at least 300 enzyme systems.

☞ DIRECTIONS: Fill a bathtub with water as hot as can be tolerated. Add 2 cups of Epsom salts. Bathe for thirty minutes, adding hot water if necessary to keep the bath water warm.

ANGELICA: Various species of angelica have been used to quiet pain by American Indians throughout North America. The European species (*Angelica archangelica*) and the Chinese species (*Angelica sinensis*) have been used in the same way in the folk medicine of Europe and China respectively. The Chinese species is sometimes sold in North America under the names dang gui or dong quai. All species contain anti-inflammatory, antispasmodic, and anodyne (pain-relieving) properties. The European species of angelica has been used in European folk medicine since antiquity, as has the Chinese species in Chinese medicine.

☞ DIRECTIONS: Place 1 tablespoon of the cut roots of either species of angelica in a pint of water and bring to a boil for two minutes in a covered pot. Remove from heat and let stand, covered, until the tea cools to room temperature. Drink the pint in 3 doses during the day.

❧ Skin ❧

■ ■ ■

The reason why treatments for skin conditions are so plentiful is because skin ailments, although usually minor as far as health risk is concerned, are so common. But skin conditions are also visible and uncomfortable and demand our attention.

Over time, useless folk remedies for the skin were smoothly weeded out— many were topical remedies, so it was usually obvious whether they worked or not. People kept the skin remedies that worked effectively and incorporated them into folk tradition.

Elsewhere in this book we cover acne, athlete's foot, bites and stings, boils and carbuncles, burns and sunburn, eczema, itching and rashes, poison ivy and poison oak, splinters, wounds and cuts, and sores and chronic skin

ulcers. In this section, we'll discuss remedies for heat rash, chapped skin, and impetigo as well as remedies designed for better overall health of the skin.

Of the conditions here, impetigo is the most serious. Impetigo is a skin condition that may be caused by Staphylococcus or Streptococcus bacteria. And, because of decades of antibiotic overuse, antibiotic-resistant strains of these bacteria are now common. It is possible, although rare, that an antibiotic-resistant strain of the bacteria might cause a systemic infection. Any infection of the skin that develops red streaks around it requires immediate medical attention.

Remedies

RED CLOVER: Red clover (*Trifolium pratense*) is a

commonly used remedy for treating skin conditions (such as acne, eczema, boils, and rashes). It can be applied externally, which is recorded in the folk traditions of Indiana, or it can be taken as a tea, which is the practice in the southern Appalachian region.

Red clover tea is also one of the most often prescribed remedies for skin conditions in professional medical herbalism in North America. Red clover was used both internally and externally for skin conditions by the Eclectic physicians at the turn of

the century. Harvey Felter, M.D., an Eclectic professor of medicine, said in his *King's American Dispensatory* that red clover, when applied externally, soothes inflamed skin, disinfects it, and promotes the growth of healthy tissue.

The plant contains more than 30 identified chemical constituents. Their properties support Felter's observations:

Besides containing antimicrobial and anti-inflammatory chemicals, red clover also contains allantoin, which promotes the healing and growth of

From the Inside Out

Some common folk remedies fall into the traditional category of "blood purifiers" (see "Blood Purifiers and Blood Builders," page 79). Traditional "blood tonic" herbs mentioned in the folk literature for skin conditions are red clover, burdock, boneset, sarsaparilla, and wild cherry bark. The idea of blood purifiers has a solid physiological basis because the skin receives all of its nutrients from the blood. Thus, these herbs are used to treat the skin "from the inside out." In the same way, toxins, allergens, or irritants in the blood can also cause symptoms of skin infection.

healthy skin tissue. Red clover has a high mineral content as well:

An ounce of the flowering tops contains one half of the minimum daily requirement of calcium, one fourth of the requirement of magnesium, and one third of the requirement of potassium. Red clover should not be used simultaneously with pharmaceutical blood-thinning medications, however, including aspirin. Taken internally, red clover may thin the blood through the actions of its coumarin constituents.

☞ DIRECTIONS: To treat the skin from the inside out, add 1 ounce of red clover tops to 1 quart of water. Simmer on the lowest possible heat until one third of the water is gone. Cool and strain. Drink the liquid in 3 doses during the day.

For external use, try this remedy from Indiana:

Scarred for Life?

Reduction or elimination of scars is a common human desire, and remedies to reduce scarring appear in several North American folk traditions. Scar formation results from wound healing or from inflammation. This natural process leaves the injured tissue stronger than it was before the injury, which helps to protect the area against repeat injury. Unfortunately, most agents that suppress scar formation, whether pharmaceutical or herbal, also tend to suppress healing. To be effective, treatments must be applied as soon as the wound is closed. Folk traditions emphasize the importance of being persistent when rubbing the oils into the skin. Coconut oil, cocoa butter, castor oil, and vitamin E oil are all used in folk medicine. Vitamin E, which is present in each of these oils, has been shown to reduce minor scarring while not suppressing healing.

Simmer whole flowering red clover plants until tender. Use just enough water to cover. Strain, press the plants into a thick mass, and sprinkle with white flour. (The flour helps add consistency to the poultice.) Place the floured poultice directly on the irritated skin. Leave on for about half an hour. You can use the red clover poultice several times a day. (The poultice can last a few days if it's kept in the refrigerator between applications.) The poultice is designed to help reduce inflammation and promote healing.

JOJOBA OIL: The Papago Indian tribe of the Southwest has used jojoba nut (*Simmondsia chinensis*) preparations to treat skin conditions such as boils and rashes. The nuts are traditionally dried and then pulverized and applied to the skin. Jojoba oil is now commercially extracted, and it is a popular addition to skin creams, oils, and ointments available in health food stores. The oil is also used today in the folk medicine of the Southwest for chapped skin.

☞ DIRECTIONS: Apply commercial jojoba oil as desired to dry, chapped skin.

PLANTAIN LEAVES: Plantain leaves (*Plantago major*) are a common weed found on lawns throughout the United States. It was naturalized in North America after the arrival of the Europeans. American Indians called it "White Man's Footprint" because it seemed to follow the European colonists wherever they went. The Delaware, Mohegan, Ojibwa, Cherokee, and other American Indian tribes used plantain for treating minor wounds and insect bites.

Plantain has been used in cultures around the world to treat wounds and skin conditions. Plantain contains a pharmacy of constituents that are beneficial to the skin, including at least 15 anti-inflammatory constituents and six analgesic chemicals. Like red clover, it contains the constituent allantoin, which promotes cell proliferation and tissue healing.

☞ DIRECTIONS: Crush a small handful of fresh plantain leaves and apply the juice locally to dry, chapped skin.

VINEGAR: Vinegar is also a remedy for chapped hands, according to folklorist Clarence Meyer's *American Folk Medicine.* The Amish use vinegar and water to treat heat rash in babies. No scientific reason for such a treatment is apparent.

☞ DIRECTIONS: After washing and drying the hands thoroughly, apply vinegar, put on a pair of gloves, and go to bed.

GARLIC PASTE: In Gypsy traditions garlic is used as a treatment for all types of skin infections, including impetigo, cuts, and wounds.

When garlic is cut or crushed, it releases a substance called allicin, one of the most potent broad-spectrum antimicrobial chemicals known. This same substance, which is part of the plant's defense system against bacteria, virus, molds, and yeast, is responsible for the burning effect of fresh cut garlic.

☞ DIRECTIONS: Pulverize 3 cloves of garlic in a blender or with a mortar and pestle. Add vinegar a drop at a time to make a thin paste that can be applied to the infected area. Apply twice a day, leaving in place for ten to fifteen minutes each time. This preparation can cause skin burns, so don't exceed the recommended time limit. Afterward, wash the area thoroughly and cover *continued on page 324*

Naturally Healthy Skin

A beautiful and youthful complexion seems always to have been highly valued, so folk tradition is filled with advice on clarifying the skin, removing blackheads and pimples, and making freckles disappear. Many of these are herbal treatments that work similarly to some of our modern over-the-counter facial products. In the Midwest, for example, the "milk" of milkweed was once used for facials. Milkweed actually secretes latex, so when the dried "milk" was peeled off the skin, it may have taken oils and blackheads with it.

Many folk treatments for the complexion seem to involve the idea of bleaching, or lightening, the skin. Although other acidic substances like tomato juice are used for this purpose, lemon juice is perhaps the most common application—it is also used to gradually bleach the hair. Cucumber pulp has also been a skin lightener in folk practice, and cucumber masks and ointments are common today in drug stores. Buttermilk is another traditional facial application that remains with us in popular complexion treatments. A little beyond buttermilk is the Midwestern advice to use sour milk that has stood at least five hours. (Mix the milk with grated horseradish and apply to the skin twice daily.) But if sour milk sounds unpleasant for a facial, it is far from the worst remedy. In the Ozarks it has been reported that a face mask of cow dung will not only clarify the complexion but also remove wrinkles! (This remedy is not recommended.) And, from the same region, it has been reported that scarring from smallpox could be prevented with the application of warm blood from a freshly killed black dog.

The most frequently reported unpleasant complexion remedy uses urine. A urine soaked diaper has been claimed as a guaranteed pimple remover in many traditions—some of these remedies specify using a boy's diaper or a girl's. More extreme is the recommendation that you drink your own urine to cure acne.

Many complexion cures do not seem to have any medical relevance, grotesque or otherwise. For example, in Europe and North America, there is a very old folk tradition that says you can rid yourself of pimples and blackheads by crawling under a bramble bush on a Friday!

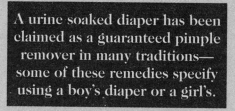

A urine soaked diaper has been claimed as a guaranteed pimple remover in many traditions— some of these remedies specify using a boy's diaper or a girl's.

To judge from the number of freckle cures found in folk tradition, these markings were once almost as despised as pimples. While some treatments aim at bleaching the skin to make the freckles fade, many remedies are magical. For example, from Georgia comes the idea that you should count your freckles, then place the same number of pebbles in a paper bag and leave the package where someone else will step on it. The person who steps on the package will get the freckles.

Water has been used magically to clear the complexion. These treatments included using water from a tree stump, water from a blacksmith's tub in which red hot metal had been plunged, water gathered on the first of June, or dew collected on the first day of May.

the area with gauze or a clean dressing.

URINE: Using your own urine as a treatment for chapped hands is part of the folklore of New England. Urine is also used for chapping in the folklore of Hispanics in the Southwest and among blacks in Louisiana. Urine therapy for cleansing wounds and treating skin infections appeared in the ancient medical systems of Mexico, Egypt, Persia, India, and China. It was used in 17th and 18th century Europe as well. Urine contains the substance urea, a disinfectant and skin moistener used in modern pharmaceutical preparations to cleanse wounds and in cosmetic products. (It is animal urine that is used in these preparations, of course.)

☞ DIRECTIONS: Apply fresh warm urine to chapped hands and skin and allow skin to air dry.

OATMEAL: Oatmeal is a treatment for chapped hands in folklorist

Clarence Meyer's collection of remedies called *American Folk Medicine*. In the method described below, oatmeal is used to both moisten and dry the skin.

☞ DIRECTIONS: Use wet oatmeal instead of soap to wash chapped hands. Then, after drying hands with a towel, rub the hands with dry oatmeal.

CLAY: Clay application is a common folk remedy for treating various skin conditions throughout the world. It was common among the North American Indians even before the arrival of the European colonists. Today, the therapeutic use of clay makes up an important part of modern Seventh Day Adventist traditions. Clay is drawing and cooling. It is most effective on moist and inflamed conditions rather than on dry, chapped skin.

☞ DIRECTIONS: Purchase bentonite clay or cosmetic grade clay at a health food store or drugstore. Mix the clay with water to make a paste and apply to the skin. Allow to dry, then gently flake off after a few hours. Wipe the clay off over a bowl. Discard the waste in your garden or on your lawn, because clay can stop up your pipes. Apply clay every few hours.

GUMWEED: Gumweed (*Grindelia spp.*) grows throughout the American Southwest and northwestern Mexico. It has been used as a skin remedy in those regions first by the American Indians and later by others who settled there.

Gumweed entered into the medical practice of the Eclectic physicians during the late 19th and early 20th centuries. In *The Eclectic Materia Medica, Pharmacology, and Therapeutics,* Harvey Felter, M.D., an Eclectic professor of medicine, states that gumweed was especially well-suited to treat those skin conditions characterized by "feeble circulation and a tendency to ulceration."

Gumweed was an official medicine in the *United States Pharmacopoeia* from 1882 until 1926. It remains an official medicine in Germany; it is used there as an expectorant for coughs. Little research has been performed into the constituents of gumweed. The resin contains anti-inflammatory constituents, so it may be useful in treating infectious or inflammatory skin conditions.

☞ DIRECTIONS: Apply the sticky sap from the leaves or flowers of gumweed to the affected areas. Reapply every few hours. Alternately, you can purchase a tincture of gumweed and use it as a wash. Reapply the tincture every few hours.

GOLDENSEAL: Goldenseal (*Hydrastis canadensis*) was used as an American Indian remedy for skin infections, such as impetigo, even before the European colonists arrived. Its use as a topical disinfectant and internal bitter tonic spread rapidly to

Salves and Ointments

Homemade salves and ointments are commonly used throughout the folklore of the world. To make one, a medicinal plant is cooked or mixed in lard, butter, beeswax, or other oily substance that remains solid at room temperature. The oily portion of the salve helps to soften and penetrate the tissues and also serves to hold the medicinal portion in place. To make a simple salve, chop, powder, crush, or grind the medicinal material as small as possible and place in the bottom of a skillet or a crock pot. Place enough lard, butter, or beeswax in the pan or pot; it should cover the plant material when melted. Leave on very lowest heat for a while—at least ten to twenty minutes for a leafy substance, forty to sixty minutes for roots. Remove from heat. Let the ointment cool to a solid state. Store lard or butter ointments in the refrigerator. Plantain, grindelia, goldenseal, rosemary, and osha are all easy to make into salves. Combinations of the herbs may make more effective salves than single herb preparations.

the English colonists in the eastern parts of the country. It has been used in one school of American medicine or another ever since. Goldenseal contains the antimicrobial substance berberine, which kills both Streptococcus and Staphylococcus bacteria, the two most common infecting agents in impetigo. Other berberine-containing plants include Oregon grape root (*Mahonia aquifolium, Berberis aquifolium*) and barberry (*Berberis vulgaris*).

☞ DIRECTIONS: Place ½ ounce of goldenseal root bark or powder in 1 pint of water. Bring to a boil, then simmer for twenty minutes. Allow the water to cool to room temperature.

Stir and, without straining, apply to the affected area with a clean cloth. Cover with a clean bandage or gauze pad. Reapply the application every two hours as desired.

ROSEMARY: Rosemary leaf *(Rosmarinus officinalis)* is a remedy from the Southwest for treating windburn and cracked and chapped skin. It is also used in that region (and other areas as well) as a wash for infectious skin conditions. The plant's leaf contains four anti-inflammatory substances—carnosol, oleanolic acid, rosmarinic acid, and ursolic acid. Rosemary also contains more than ten antiseptic constituents.

☞ DIRECTIONS: Crush some rosemary leaves and warm in a pan on low heat. Add some lard to make a salve. Simmer over low heat until the lard takes on the color and aroma of the rosemary. Let cool. Apply to the affected areas as desired.

Alternately, place 1 ounce of crushed rosemary leaf in a 1-pint jar and fill with boiling water. Cover tightly and let stand until the water reaches room temperature. Apply as a wash to the affected area, using a clean cloth, as often as desired.

WATERMELON RIND: To treat rash in babies, the Amish suggest rubbing the affected area with watermelon rind.

☞ DIRECTIONS: Rub the affected area with the inside of a watermelon rind. Be sure to dry the area thoroughly and apply a talcum powder or some other drying agent.

OSHA: Osha *(Ligusticum porteri),* which is native to the Rocky Mountains, was a panacea to the American Indians in the area. The plant remains one of the most important folk remedies of the residents of the upper Rio Grande Valley. Osha is used for colds, flu, bronchitis, and also as a skin wash for superficial infections.

Very little scientific research has been performed into either the constituents or the pharmaceutical properties of the plant, but a close Chinese relative of the plant (*Ligusticum wallichi*) has been studied extensively. The main constituent of its aromatic oil is alpha-pinene, which has antimicrobial and disinfectant properties. Constituents called ligustilides, which are common to both the North American and Chinese species, have broad spectrum antibiotic effects as well as antiviral and antifungal properties.

☞ DIRECTIONS: Using a coffee grinder, grind a piece of osha root into a powder. Spread the powder in a small skillet. Add enough lard or butter to cover the powder when

Sweating It Out

Many traditional folk remedies are called diaphoretics—plants or foods that make you sweat. Constituents in these plants increase the blood circulation to the skin, which, when taken internally, can be helpful in healing various skin conditions. Some diaphoretics are recommended for common skin ailments in the folklore of the southern Appalachian mountains. For example, burdock, boneset, elder flowers, and yarrow have all been used in folklore there to treat skin conditions "from the inside out" by increasing circulation to the skin.

melted. Put on low heat until the lard or butter is melted. Stir well and let stand at room temperature until the salve becomes solid. To treat a skin infection, apply the salve to the skin every three hours.

Alternately, mix the osha with enough honey to make a paste. Apply to a piece of gauze and use a bandage to hold in place over the affected area. Osha may irritate the skin. If this occurs, reduce the frequency of the treatments or try another remedy.

CORNSTARCH AND CORNMEAL: Cornstarch and cornmeal are common agents used to treat moist skin conditions such as heat rash, according to folklorist Clarence Meyer's *American Folk Medicine.* Cornstarch and cornmeal are also used to treat chapped skin and prickly heat. Cornstarch "dusting powder" appears in the contemporary folklore of Indiana.

☞ DIRECTIONS: Wash the area, wipe it dry, and dust with cornstarch.

VITAMIN E OIL: Vitamin E oil rubbed into scar tissue will help to reduce a scar, according to the traditions of the Amish. The Amish also use cocoa butter and castor oil for the same purpose. All three oils contain vitamin E, but the vitamin E oil contains higher amounts. Vitamin E has been shown to reduce scarring in a variety of scientific experiments. Treatment with vitamin E for skin grafts after severe burns did not work in one trial, however, so there may be a limit as to what can be accomplished with this remedy.

☞ DIRECTIONS: As soon as possible after a wound is closed, rub vitamin E oil (or one of the other oils above) into the tissues for five to ten minutes twice a day. The rubbing, which increases circulation and can break up deep scars, is an important part of the application process. Continue rubbing in the oil on a daily basis for months if necessary, or at least until improvement appears.

POTATO POULTICE: According to folk traditions of the Gypsies, a potato poultice will improve puffy skin, espe-
continued on page 333

329

Unconventional Wart Cures

Warts are infectious growths in the outer layers of the skin. They are contagious and can spread from person to person. Most warts are not health-threatening, but they can be a nuisance, and most who have them are eager to get rid of them.

One of folk medicine's most bizarre wart cures involves graveyards, not crossroads, however. In the southern and western United States, according to folklorists, some residents attempt to cure warts by taking a dead cat to a graveyard at midnight. (Whether or not the cat is killed for this purpose is not always specified in the folk literature.) When a noise is heard, the cat is thrown in the direction of the sound. In Tennessee, people believe the sound heard is the devil—"coming to get his people." As the person throws the cat, he or she must say, "Cat follow the devil, warts follow the cat."

Wart cures are a popular part of folk medicine. That's probably because warts have plagued humanity for centuries. In ancient times, people weren't sure where warts came from, so they invented causes for the malady. For example, the belief that warts were caused by touching toads is probably due to the similarity between a wart's appearance and a toad's lumpy, wartlike skin.

Today, we know warts are caused by the human papilloma virus (HPV). Scientists once thought warts were caused by just one kind of virus; now we know there are at least 60 types of HPVs that cause a wide variety of warts, from plantar warts that grow on the feet to the warts that most often appear on the hands and fingers. Warts can

Wart Cures

There are some wart cures that are gruesome as well as dangerous. Many of these cures require the use of blood, either drawn from the wart or applied to it. In one remedy, blood drawn from a wart by repeatedly pricking it with a pin is to be put on grains of corn that are then fed to chickens. (Presumably the chicken then gets the warts—but perhaps not before the sufferer gets an infection!) In another remedy, warm bloody meat from a freshly killed hog is applied directly to the wart. Finally, one remedy suggests rubbing the wart with the head of a recently killed cock; the cock is then buried under the eaves of your home or barn.

emerge anywhere on the skin including the genital and anal areas, and even internally.

Some wart cures seem medicinal, like those that require the use of dandelion or milkweed juice. Other treatments appear ritualistic: A treatment from North Carolina instructs patients to gather seven different kinds of leaves, rub each on the wart twice, and bury the leaves where no one will find them. But most folk cures have a magical element. Take, for instance, the blacksmith's water cure. Water into which a blacksmith has plunged his hot iron has an ancient reputation as a magical remedy for many things. Iron supposedly had supernatural properties, so a blacksmith's water was therefore thought to be magical. Iron has long been used in the folk traditions of many cultures.

Why are wart cures so popular? Probably because they seem to work. Even if left alone, most warts will disappear on their own in a few months. By the time a person is annoyed enough with a wart to seek a remedy, the wart is

Unwelcome Warts

Many magical wart cures are uncharitable to say the least, especially when they involve the intent of giving the warts to someone else. This sort of behavior can be illustrated in a cure that requires an individual to rub his warts with a penny and leave the penny in the road—whoever picks up the penny is believed to take the warts along with him!

▩   ▩   ▩

probably already in its final stages and it will soon disappear. Most folk cures capitalize on this fact. One cure from the southern United States says to rub warts with the sole of a shoe. As the leather wears away, so will the warts. A cure from Pennsylvania directs the patient to put a chalk mark for each wart on the back of an old iron wood-burning stove. When the chalk marks wear away, the warts will be gone. In both of these cases, the remedies are likely to work—simply because of patience and the passage of time.

Cures for warts often involve physical contact with certain items. Similar cures call for rubbing the wart with a potato, onion, or dish rag. The item used to rub the wart is then hidden in a place where it will decay; for example, under the eaves of a house. If a dishrag is the chosen item, the remedy often specifies that the dish rag be stolen from the individual's mother. (Children tend to acquire warts more often than adults.)

There is little evidence that some of these cures actually have the medical ability to cure warts. More likely, it is the power of suggestion—and the passage of time—that is so successful in curing warts. For these reasons, many ancient wart cures continue to be practiced and passed from one generation to the next.

cially those "bags" under the eyes. This same method is taught in contemporary naturopathic medical schools to reduce inflammation of the skin.

☞ DIRECTIONS: Thoroughly clean 2 or 3 potatoes. Grate (including the potato skins) and press them with your hands into a paste. Apply to the affected areas of the skin. Leave in place while relaxing for fifteen minutes. Remove the poultice and clean and dry the area.

MILK: Milk is applied to the skin to relieve the irritation and discomfort of a variety of skin ailments in the folklore of the Hispanic Southwest. The remedy is also popular in the folk medicine of New England. In the southern Appalachians, it is buttermilk that's preferred. These remedies traditionally used whole milk right from the cow, which, these days, is not usually available for sale. If you're going to try this remedy, use whole milk, not low fat milk. The short- and medium-chain fatty acids in the butterfat of whole milk may have a mild antimicrobial effect on the skin. Any beneficial effect of this remedy is more likely due to the soothing quality of the milk rather than any actual pharmaceutical activity.

☞ DIRECTIONS: Wash the affected area with milk or buttermilk as desired.

MUNG BEAN PASTE: A treatment for heat rash or prickly heat from Chinese folklore is mung bean "soap," which is made from a mixture of cooked mung beans and sugar. The most important component of the formula may be the sugar, however, because by nature it is drying and cooling. Sugar has been used in various cultures to cleanse wounds. The astringent properties of the beans may also have a beneficial effect.

☞ DIRECTIONS: Cook mung beans until they can be mashed into the consistency of a paste. Add enough sugar so that the beans are sweet to the taste. Apply to the affected area, rubbing as if the paste were soap. Leave the paste in place for fifteen minutes. Then remove, dry the area well, and dust with talcum powder or another drying agent.

Sore Throat

A sore throat is a painful irritation in the throat. A sore throat can range from mild scratchiness to severe pain and difficulty in swallowing.

A sore throat is most frequently seen as a symptom of a virus. When an individual suffers from a common cold, the nasal passages are congested and the person is forced to breathe through the mouth, leaving the throat dry and irritated. Coughing may also irritate the throat, as will the secretions that drain into the throat from the back of the nose during a cold.

A severe sore throat may be caused by a bacterial (usually *Streptococcus* bacteria, or strep) infection of the throat, middle ear, or sinuses. It is difficult to determine from the symptoms whether a sore throat is due to a virus or to strep (although a doctor can tell the difference using laboratory tests). Both infections may be accompanied by fever, headache, and fatigue, and both infections normally get better on their own. The fever subsides within a few days, the sore throat improves, and all signs of infection are usually gone within two weeks.

The complications of strep throat begin between one and six weeks after the first appearance of the sore throat, usually after about two weeks. For this reason, any sore throat that lasts more than a week requires a visit to the doctor. A number of individuals who carry Streptococcus bacteria are without any symptoms at all. In fact, 15 to 20 percent of children are carriers, and most are asymptomatic. Concern for complications comes only with active inflammation, although the symptoms may seem minor.

Strep throat can have serious complications, however. A prolonged strep infection can result in damage to the heart (called rheumatic fever) or to the kidneys. These complications are rare, however— less than 1 percent of strep throats result in these illnesses. But the complications are common enough to warrant antibiotic prescriptions for strep infections, which is the standard treatment in modern medicine. Antibiotics for strep also reduce secondary infections, such as ear infection or pneumonia, that might accompany the sore throat.

(Antibiotics are of no value in sore throats caused by viruses.)

Folk remedy treatments for sore throats fall into five categories. First, there are remedies that act as astringents, which reduce swelling of the mucous membrane tissues and thereby reduce pain. Second, there are demulcents such as slippery elm. These herbs or foods have a slimy constituency that is soothing to inflamed tissues. The third category contains plants used to treat sore throat like goldenseal or garlic that are antibacterial and antiviral. In the fourth category are the remedies such as mint and echinacea that contain local anesthetics that help numb a sore throat. Finally, many of the herbs used in folk remedies for sore throat contain anti-inflammatory constituents that may reduce pain and swelling. Most of the remedies combine more than one of these actions. For example, sage leaf is both astringent and antiseptic. Mint is both antiseptic and anesthetic. Willow bark is both astringent and anti-inflammatory. Most folk remedies call for gargling the substance, and most can be swallowed after gargling for further benefits.

Remedies

SLIPPERY ELM: Slippery elm bark (*Ulmus spp., Ulmus fulva*) was used to treat sore throats by members of at least six American Indian tribes, including the Iroquois and the Cherokee, even before the arrival of the European colonists. Slippery elm has been a folkloric treatment for sore throat in the United States at least since the early 1800s when its use was popularized by the Thomsonian herbalists. Slippery elm was an official remedy in the *United States Pharmacopoeia* from 1820 until 1930. Slippery elm throat lozenges have been sold throughout the United States since the late 1800s. They

are available today in many health food stores and pharmacies. Slippery elm powder, when moistened, has a slimy quality that is soothing to inflamed mucous membranes. Professional medical herbalists in the United States, Australia, and Europe use slippery elm to soothe inflammations of the mouth, throat, and intestines. Its use continues today in the folk medicine of New England, North Carolina, and Indiana.

☞ DIRECTIONS: Place 1 tablespoon of powdered slippery elm bark in a cup. Fill with boiling water. Let steep for ten minutes. Stir, without straining, and first gargle, then swallow ½-cup doses to soothe a sore throat. Do this as often as desired. Alternately, make honey lozenges of slippery elm by mixing the slippery elm powder with hot honey. Spread the paste on a marble slab or other nonstick surface coated with sugar or cornstarch. With a rolling pin, roll the mixture flat to about the thickness of a pancake. Sprinkle with sugar and cornstarch. With a knife, cut into small, separate squares. Or pinch off pieces and roll into ¼-inch balls. Flatten the balls into round lozenges. Allow lozenges to air-dry in a well-ventilated area for twelve hours. Then store them in the refrigerator. Suck on lozenges to help heal sore throats.

Also, the most basic method, mentioned in several folk traditions, is to chew on the bark and swallow the juice or suck on the plain bark powder.

RED ROOT: Red root (*Ceanothus americanus, Ceanothus spp.*) was used for a wide variety of ailments, including colds and coughs, by American Indians living in the regions where it grows. Eclectic and Physiomedicalist physicians adopted the use of red root in the mid-19th century. A tea of the leaves was used during the Civil War as a treatment for malaria. Today, red root is used to treat sore throats in the folk medicine of Appalachia and by Hispanics in the Southwest.

Red root is astringent like black tea and was even used as a substitute for tea during the Civil War when black tea was unavailable. Some Ceanothus species contain a small amount of caffeine. Red root also contains anti-inflammatory and antimicrobial constituents that may help soothe and disinfect a sore throat. Its constituents ceanothic acid and ceanothetric acid have specifically shown to inhibit the growth of Streptococcus bacteria in laboratory experiments. (A tincture must be used, rather than a tea, to take advantage of the anti-streptococcal activity, however.) Red root has not been tested in clinical trials. The tea is a better source of the astringent constituents than the tincture and is the form used by physicians during the last century.

☞ DIRECTIONS: Simmer 1 ounce of red root in 1 pint of water on low heat for twenty minutes. Let cool to room temperature. Gargle doses of 1 tablespoon and swallow, four times a day. Alternately, you can purchase a tincture of red root at a health food store or herb shop. Hold a teaspoon dose of the tincture in the mouth and swish it around. Then gargle and swallow. Do this four times a day for as long as necessary.

GOLDENSEAL: Goldenseal (*Hydrastis canadensis*) was a sore throat remedy among eastern American Indian tribes. The colonists quickly adopted the plant as a household medicine, and by the 1830s physicians were using it to treat sore throats. Goldenseal was an official medicine in the *United States Pharmacopoeia* from 1840 until 1920. It is still used today to treat sore throats in the folk medicine of North Carolina.

The plant's constituent berberine is a strong antibiotic—about as potent as pharmaceutical drugs of the sulfa group. Berberine must come in direct contact with microorganisms in order to kill them, and it does not enter the bloodstream the way most pharmaceutical antibiotics do. Oregon grape root (*Mahonia aquifolium, Berberis aquifolium*) and barberry (*Berberis vulgaris*) also contain berberine. (Both plants were used for treating sore throats by American Indians in the regions where the plants grow.) Of the three plants, goldenseal is probably best for treating sore throats because, unlike the other two plants, it contains power-ful astringents. However, goldenseal is now an endangered species and is very expensive. Oregon grape root and barberry root, on the other hand, are inexpensive and plentiful.

☞ DIRECTIONS: Place 1 ounce of one of the above roots in a pint of water. Bring to a boil and simmer on the lowest heat for twenty minutes. Let cool to room temperature. Gargle and swallow doses of 1 to 2 tablespoons three to four times a day.

HOREHOUND: A folk remedy for sore throats from contemporary Indiana is horehound (*Marrubium vulgare*). Horehound has been used in European folk medicine since the time of the ancient Greeks. It was later used for treating sore throats in this country by the Mahuna and Navaho Indian tribes. Horehound became an official cough remedy in the *United States Pharmacopoeia* between 1840 and 1910. It remains an approved medicine for coughs by the German government today.

The herb is most famous as a cough medicine. Horehound cough drops are available in some health food stores and pharmacies. Besides its expectorant properties, horehound also contains astringent tannins (like those in tea) and anti-inflammatory and antimicrobial aromatic oils.

☞ DIRECTIONS: Place 1 tablespoon of dried horehound in a cup and fill with boiling water. Cover and let steep for fifteen minutes. Strain and sweeten with honey. Gargle ½-cup doses as desired.

LICORICE: A folk remedy from China for sore throats is licorice tea. Licorice is used as a medicine in every major traditional medical system in the world. Extracts of licorice were originally used to make licorice candy, but the spice anise is used for that purpose today. Licorice was an official medicine in the *United States Pharma-*

copoeia from 1820 until 1975; it was listed as a flavoring agent and a demulcent and expectorant for cough syrups.

Licorice root has a sweet flavor and a soothing demulcent quality. It also contains anti-inflammatory constituents similar to steroid drugs. (These constituents act systemically; that is, after the licorice has been digested. These constituents are therefore unlikely to account for any soothing topical effect of the licorice tea.) The following method of preparing the tea comes from Chinese folklore.

☞ DIRECTIONS: Place ½ ounce of licorice root in 1 quart of water. Boil on low heat in an uncovered pot until half the water has evaporated. Drink the remaining pint in 2 doses during the course of a day. Repeat for up to three days. Don't take licorice if you are taking steroid drugs.

OAK BARK: Oak bark *(Quercus spp.)* has been used to treat sore throats since antiquity in European folk medicine. In this country, oak bark was used for the same purpose by members of the Delaware, Cherokee, Houma, Alabama, and Iroquois Indian tribes. Later, from 1820 until 1930, oak bark was an official medicine in the *United States Pharmacopoeia*.

Oak bark contains a high level of tannins—the same substances found in black tea. Oak bark is mentioned today in the folk medicine of North Carolina. It is also used by professional medical herbalists in North America and Europe.

☞ DIRECTIONS: Boil 3 tablespoons of oak bark in 1 pint of water for twenty minutes. Let cool to room temperature and strain. Gargle with 1 or 2 tablespoons of the tea three to four times a day for as long as necessary.

ROSE: A sore throat remedy in the Hispanic folklore of the Southwest is a tea of rose petals *(Rosa spp.)*. Rose petals have also been used by American

Indians of the Costanoan, Skagut, and Snohomish tribes to treat throat problems. In addition, rose petals are among the top ten of the most often prescribed herbs in contemporary Arabic medicine.

The petals have a strong astringent action and can tone up swollen and inflamed mucous membranes, which is their chief medicinal use in Arabic medicine. The rose oil that gives the flowers their scent also contains antimicrobial and anti-inflammatory substances. The petals are considered to be "cooling" in Arabic medicine, indicating that clinical anti-inflammatory effects have been observed in their medical traditions.

☞ DIRECTIONS: Pour 1 pint of boiling water over a handful of rose petals in a 1-pint jar. Cover well to retain the aromatic oils, and let stand until the water reaches room temperature. Gargle ½-cup doses as desired for sore throat. Avoid commercial roses and roses that have been sprayed with strong pesticides.

HERBAL STEAM: An entry in folklorist Clarence Meyer's collection of remedies, called *American Folk Medicine,* suggests inhaling steam from an herbal tea to treat severely painful sore throats. The herbs included are sage *(Salvia officinalis),* boneset *(Eupatorium perfoliatum),* catnip *(Nepeta cataria),* hop *(Humulus lupulus),* and horehound *(Marrubium vulgare).* The mixture contains anti-inflammatory aromatic oils that presumably can rise with the steam and affect the throat. The steam itself may be antiviral. Most of the viruses that infect the mucous membranes cannot survive at temperatures equal to those in the body's core—about 98.6°F. Thus, the viruses remain at the cooler membranes, near the surface of the body (in the mucous membranes of the respiratory tract). Inhaling hot steam may kill the viruses on contact.

☞ DIRECTIONS: Place a handful each of sage, boneset, catnip, hop, and horehound in a large bowl. Pour 1 quart of boiling water over the herbs and inhale the steam that rises, being careful not to burn yourself. If you don't have one or two of the herbs in the formula, use the ones mentioned that you do have.

OSHA: Osha (*Ligusticum porteri*), a Rocky Mountain plant, was used for a variety of ailments by American Indians living in that region. Osha remains one of the most important folk remedies of American Indians and Hispanic residents of the upper Rio Grande Valley in New Mexico and Colorado. A traditional herbalist of the area, Michael Moore, recommends the tea below for sore throat. Osha contains disinfectant aromatic oils and local anesthetic aromatic oils. One of its constituents has antibacterial and antiviral properties.

☞ DIRECTIONS: Grind an osha root in a coffee grinder. Place 1 teaspoon of the powder in a cup and fill with boiling water. Cover tightly and allow to stand until the water reaches room temperature. Gargle ¼- to ½-cup doses as desired.

Alternately, mix the powdered osha with enough hot honey to make a paste. Roll the paste into balls as big around as dimes. Store the balls in the refrigerator, where they will cool to a more solid consistency. Suck on the lozenges for sore throat. You can do this as often as desired.

MINT: Both the Chinese and the Paiute Indians used mint teas (*Mentha spp.*) when treating sore throats. Mint contains a number of anti-inflammatory, antimicrobial, and local anesthetic constituents. The eight anesthetic constituents it contains may provide immediate (but temporary) relief from the pain of sore throat.

☞ DIRECTIONS: Place 1 ounce of peppermint leaves in a 1-pint jar and fill with boiling water. Cover tightly and let the tea cool to room temperature, shaking the bottle from time to time to mix the contents. Gargle ½-cup doses of the tea as desired.

VINEGAR: To treat a sore throat, Indiana folklore advises a gargle with vinegar. Another tradition suggests alternating vinegar gargles with saltwater gargles. Most microorganisms cannot live in an acid medium. Vinegar is a weak acid, so it may kill the infectious organisms. Salt also kills some microorganisms.

☞ DIRECTIONS: Gargle with straight vinegar two times a day. Wait ten minutes after the vinegar gargle and gargle with salt water. To make the saltwater gargle, add 1 teaspoon of salt to 1 cup of hot water and mix. Gargle as often as desired.

WILLOW: Willow bark (*Salix spp.*) is used as an astringent gargle for sore throats in the Hispanic folk medicine of the Southwest. The same method has been used by the Cherokee and Iroquois Indians and also by the Alaskan Eskimos. Willow bark is astringent. It also contains aspirinlike compounds that may help reduce a fever.

☞ DIRECTIONS: Simmer 3 tablespoons of willow bark in 1 pint of water for twenty to thirty minutes. Gargle with ½-cup doses as desired throughout the day as often as necessary.

COLD COMPRESS: A hydrotherapy treatment from North Carolina folklore calls for applying a cold wet compress to the throat and covering it with a dry one. The method is also used in the Seventh Day Adventist healing tradition. The treatment has its roots in the nature cure and hydrotherapy traditions of Germany, brought to North America by German immigrants near the turn of the 20th century.

☞ DIRECTIONS: Soak a cotton cloth in cold water. Wring it out and wrap it around the front of the neck below the ears. Be careful to avoid chilling the back of the neck. Wrap a warm wool scarf around the cold cloth and lie down. The cold cloth will supposedly attract circulation to the area, which in turn promotes healing of the throat. The body will usually heat the cold cloth in twenty to forty minutes. Repeat the treatment two to four times each day.

ONION SYRUP: Here's a recipe from New England for onion syrup that is remarkably similar to a recipe from North Carolina. The New England recipe calls for sliced raw onions to be placed in a bowl and covered with sugar. Allow the onion to stand until a syrup forms. Adding water is not necessary because the sugar draws the onion juice out of the onions. (It may take a day or two for the syrup to form, however.) The method used in North Carolina is similar, but the onion-and-sugar mixture is placed in a baking pan and baked in the oven until the syrup forms. (Baking presumably speeds up the process.) The onions contain antimicrobial substances, which attack the organisms that are causing the infection. These substances are the same ones that give an onion its odor, and they are also responsible for the burning sensation your eyes feel after you slice an onion.

☞ DIRECTIONS: Fill a bowl or baking pan with raw onions. Pour enough sugar over them to cover. Then, either let them stand or bake them on medium heat, depending on how fast you need the syrup. Take the syrup in single tablespoon doses as often as desired.

GARLIC: Both the Amish and the Seventh Day Adventists, two religious groups that advocate natural remedies, suggest sucking on a garlic lozenge to treat a sore throat. Garlic, when sliced or crushed, releases the antimicrobial substance allicin. Allicin kills many bacteria, including strep, and some viruses. Seventh Day Adventists Agatha Thrash, M.D., and Calvin Thrash, M.D., in their book *Home Remedies: Hydrotherapy, Massage, Charcoal, and Other Simple Treatments,* say that sore throats sometimes disappear within a few hours of using this technique.

☞ DIRECTIONS: Slice a garlic clove down the middle and place a half clove on each side of the mouth, between the teeth and cheeks. Suck on the cloves like lozenges.

MYRRH GUM: Myrrh gum *(Commiphora myrrha)* has been used as a disinfectant in the Mediterranean region since the time of the ancient Egyptians. Its use spread to India, China, and Europe along Arab trade routes. Its use as a disinfectant was popularized throughout the eastern United States by the Thomsonian herbalists of the early 1800s. Myrrh gum is a powerful antiseptic, and it is also astringent—both properties are beneficial to a throat infection.

☞ DIRECTIONS: Purchase some myrrh gum tincture at a health food store or herb shop. Add 1 teaspoon to ¼ cup of hot water and use as a gargle.

HOT WATER GARGLE: The Seventh Day Adventists advise a hot water gargle for a sore throat. The viruses most often responsible for sore throats cannot survive at temperatures above normal body temperature. If you gargle with hot water, it will come in contact with the throat's membranes, raising the continued on page 349

Patent Medicines

※ ※ ※

From colonial times until the early 20th century the drug industry was a free-for-all. Effective drugs that were available competed with all sorts of panaceas that ranged from useless to dangerous. In this wild marketplace, patent medicine vendors were advertising pioneers.

At first, prepackaged remedies were imported, but after the Revolution, American entrepreneurs made and marketed their own medicines. Hundreds of hopeful medicine-makers took out patents for their compounds but couldn't compete with the advertising budgets of those who were successful. The heavy trend in promotion accelerated through the century and was boosted by the Civil War—from which many soldiers returned addicted to bottled medicines. The war also expanded the audience for newspapers, which soon became heavily subsidized by medicine accounts. When the price of newsprint rose, marketers turned to almanacs, handbills, and, above all, the outdoors—where buildings, boulders, and whole hillsides were emblazoned with their products' names.

Salesmanship reached fever pitch in the "medicine shows" of the 1880s. There the product was secondary to entertainment. The Kickapoo Indian Medicine Company, for instance, might have 75 shows touring the country at one time. Founded by three white men, it employed American Indians to enact dire scenarios from which they were saved by a medicine called Kickapoo Indian Saqwa. The sales team for Hamlin's Wizard Oil included a singing quartet. William Rockefeller (John D. Rockefeller's father) used his talents as marksman, ventriloquist, and hypnotist to attract Midwest crowds to his medicinal products. Other salesmen posed as Quakers, Shakers, and Oriental

Medicine from Around the World

Snake oil has indeed been used in homemade medicines, along with goose grease, rabbit lard, polecat grease, and skunk oil. Patent medicines generally strove for a more exotic appeal. Besides alleged American Indian sources, far-flung locales were evoked. Dr. Lin's Celestial Balm of China, Bragg's Arctic Liniment, Hayne's Arabian Ointment, Jayne's Spanish Alternative, and Druid Ointment ("handed down from mystic days when Stonehenge was a busy temple") were just a few choices. Household remedies tended to be specific ("For rheumatism, apply oil from a cooked snake on the sore area") but commercial ones were notorious cure-alls. Helmbold's Extract of Buchu claimed to help at least 21 separate ailments from "confused ideas" to "paralysis of the organs of generation."

mystics—whatever it took to move the goods. Many "doctors" and "professors" were addicted to their own wares, which sometimes contained alcohol, opium, chloroform, or cocaine. (Other products were not so dangerous. They contained colored water or candy, like Princess Lotus Blossom's Vital Sparks.)

Snake oil, which was actually fat rendered from a snake, was among the top-selling medicines of the time. The product was used to treat a variety of ills, from arthritis to earache. Ingredients in a bottle of snake oil usually included the oil, but it could also include anything but the oil. Thus, throughout the history of the U.S. patent medicine industry, the terms "snake oil" and "snake oil salesman" have been used to describe any dubious product and its seller.

Snake oil really was among the nostrums flooding the land. But why was it singled out to represent all the bogus products? Classic associations, like the serpent in the garden, probably helped. Contemporary emblems were likely the key, however. The perennially popular Swaim's Panacea bore a label depicting Hercules battling the many-headed snakelike Hydra. On the label for Dr. Hostetter's Celebrated Stomachic Bitters Tonic, a naked St. George slays the fabled dragon. In 1905, writer Samuel Hopkins Adams published two series of articles in Collier's magazine—one on patent medicines and the other on medical quacks. In his exposé, he attacked 264 companies and individuals by name, exposing their involvement in drug sales that were dangerous and addictive. The American Medical Association then distributed 150,000 copies of

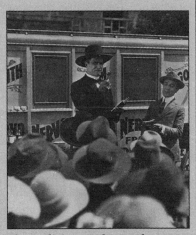

The medicine vendors and customers of days gone by.

Adams' "The Great American Fraud." This action marked the beginning of the end for unregulated drug sales. In 1906, Congress passed the Pure Food and Drug Act, which was the beginning of federal regulation. Ironically, consumption of patent medicines increased after the Pure Food and Drug Act of 1906, because with the worst products off the market, those remaining were believed to be safe.

temperature there and killing the viruses. Hot water also draws blood circulation to the area, which increases the natural immune response to the infection.

☞ DIRECTIONS: Gargle with water as hot as you can stand.

SALTWATER GARGLE: An Indiana sore throat remedy is the saltwater gargle. Salt is astringent and antimicrobial, so it may relieve pain while attacking the organisms causing the infection.

☞ DIRECTIONS: Add 1 teaspoon of salt to a cup of hot water, mix, and use as a gargle as often as desired.

LEMON: An Indiana folk tradition for curing a sore throat suggests sucking on a lemon that has been sprinkled with salt. A Gypsy version of the same treatment calls for lemon juice and salt diluted with water. Lemon is naturally acidic. Salt increases the lemon's acidity through a chemical reaction that forms dilute hydrochloric acid, which is even more acidic than lemon juice is alone. Many microorganisms are killed by weak acids, so this strong Gypsy gargle may indeed kill infectious organisms.

☞ DIRECTIONS: To use the Gypsy method, juice a whole lemon into a bowl and add a pinch of sea salt. Add 1 teaspoon of the concentrated lemon-salt mixture to 1 cup of water. Gargle some solution three to four times a day as often as necessary.

ECHINACEA: Echinacea (*Echinacea angustifolia*) was used by the Plains Indians for a wide variety of infectious diseases. The Cheyenne, Comanche, and Kiowa all used the herb to treat sore throats. Constituents in the angustifolia species can offer some relief from sore throat pain by producing a tingling and numbness in the mouth and throat that can last for more than half an hour. (These local anesthetic effects are not present in *Echinacea purpurea,* the species used in most of the commercial echinacea products, however. The root or powder of the *Echinacea angustifolia* species is sometimes available, however.) In addition, echinacea is an immune stimulant. It may help the body fight the infection that is causing the sore throat.

☞ DIRECTIONS: Obtain whole or chopped *Echinacea angustifolia* root at a health food store or herb shop. Grind a small amount in a coffee grinder. Stir ½ teaspoon of the powder into 2 ounces of warm water. Gargle the water, powder and all, for as long as you can, allowing the powder to coat your throat and mouth.

SAGE LEAF: Another sore throat remedy from Indiana is sage tea (*Salvia officinalis*), which is made from the common kitchen spice. Sage is a strong astringent, and it also contains anti-inflammatory and antimicrobial aromatic oils. Cultivated garden sage has been used as a medicine in the Mediterranean region since the time of the ancient Egyptians. It is a common remedy for sore throat in the professional medical herbalism of Europe and North America. It is an approved medicine for sore throats in Germany.

☞ DIRECTIONS: Place 1 tablespoon of sage leaf in a cup and fill with boiling water. Cover and let stand until it reaches room temperature. Gargle ¼-cup doses three to four times a day for a sore throat for as long as necessary. The concentrated essential oil of sage and the alcohol tincture should not be taken during pregnancy.

❦ Sores and Chronic ❧ Skin Ulcers

■ ■ ■

Sores, called skin ulcers in medical terminology, are localized sore spots on the body where the tissues are ruptured or abraded. These sores may result from a slow-healing wound or other trauma to the skin, acute bacterial infections, chronic bacterial and fungal infections, or rare systemic diseases. Bedsores, called decubitus or trophic ulcers, can be caused by pressure from a bed, wheelchair, or other constant source of stress on the bony parts of the body. (Bedsores tend to occur in the bedridden, paralyzed, or chronically incapacitated patients.) Poor circulation to the skin, malnutrition, chronic infection, and deficient immune response all play a part in the chronic

nature of skin ulcers as well.

Most folk remedies combine disinfecting and circulatory-stimulating properties to treat sores. Others provide soothing, protective coatings for the sores. Note that sores that accompany nerve damage, such as may occur in paralysis or diabetes, must be treated only with medical supervision. Some of the herbs and remedies in this section can cause burns to the skin or skin irritation, so individuals with impaired sensory nerves should not use them; they may not realize that their skin is becoming inflamed.

Remedies

GARLIC: A remedy from contemporary Appalachia

for treating sores is garlic (*Allium sativum*). Garlic is also recorded as a treatment for skin infection in contemporary Gypsy folklore. When garlic is crushed, it releases allicin, a potent broad-spectrum antimicrobial agent. Allicin protects the plant against infection by bacteria, viruses, molds, yeast, and fungi. It will also kill these organisms in laboratory dishes or in open wounds. Allicin breaks down into other substances within a few days, so disinfectant garlic preparations should be made fresh. Fresh garlic can cause serious skin burns, however, and should never be left in contact with the skin for more than 20 to 25 minutes. The use of garlic can be especially risky for patients who have neurological conditions.

Garlic can irritate the skin, and these individuals may not be able to feel the garlic's burning sensation. For this reason, they should use garlic with care or avoid using it altogether.

☞ DIRECTIONS: Crush 3 cloves of garlic with a mortar and pestle, or blend the cloves in a blender. Mix with an equal volume of hot honey. Allow to stand until the honey reaches room temperature, mixing occasionally. Apply the mixture to the ulcer with a piece of gauze. Then remove and wash the area thoroughly after ten to fifteen minutes. Repeat the treatment three to four times a day.

GOLDENSEAL: In the early 1800s, American botanist Constantine Rafinesque traveled throughout the Ohio and the upper Mississippi River Valley, investigating the American Indians' use of local plants. He eventually published *Medical Flora* in 1830, one of the first books on the botany of North American plants. In the book he described a plant called "yellow puccoon," which we now know as goldenseal (*Hydrastis canadensis*). Rafinesque noted that the American Indians made a powder of goldenseal and used it to treat ulcers and slow-healing wounds.

Goldenseal rapidly entered into medical practice in North America and has been used ever since by one medical discipline or another. Goldenseal contains the antimicrobial substance berberine, which kills a broad spectrum of bacteria, viruses, yeast, and molds. In the folklore of Appalachia, a tea of goldenseal is recommended as a wash for skin ulcers. Although some Appalachians can still find goldenseal growing underfoot, it is now an endangered species and may soon be unavailable in stores. Other berberine-containing plants such as Oregon grape root (*Mahonia aquifolium*) or barberry (*Berberis vulgaris*) make good substitutes.

☞ DIRECTIONS: Place ½ ounce of goldenseal root bark or powder (or use one of the other herbs, noted) in a pint of water. Bring the water to a boil, then simmer for twenty minutes. Allow to cool to room temperature. Stir and, without straining, apply the tea to the affected area with a clean cloth. Do not wipe off, just cover with a clean bandage or gauze pad. Apply the tea every two hours. Simultaneously, drink 2-ounce doses of the tea two to four times a day.

HONEY: Since the dawn of medical history, honey has been used around the world as a folk remedy to disinfect wounds and burns. Honey appears today in the folk literature of the Amish, Hispanics in the Southwest, Chinese immigrants, and residents of Indiana.

Honey, because it is naturally dehydrated, attracts water. When applied to an ulcer, honey draws fluid out of the tissues, which simultaneously cleanses the sore. Thus, most infectious microorganisms cannot live in the presence of honey, because the honey literally sucks the fluid right out of them. Physicians in India experimented with honey-gauze dressings for treating burns and found that the honey applications had stronger antibiotic effects than silver sulfadiazine, the most common antibiotic dressing used for burns. The burns of the honey-treated patients also healed faster. What's more, the honey offered greater relief of pain and reduced scarring as well.

☞ DIRECTIONS: Apply honey to a piece of sterile gauze and place directly on the ulcer. Hold in place with tape. Change the honey dressing three or four times a day.

CHAPARRAL: Chaparral (*Larrea tridentata*) is a popular remedy of the American Indians of the Southwest. It is most commonly used by tribes in that area as a wash to treat various skin conditions. Chaparral has a powerful odor, and its aromatic constituents, which include alpha-pinene, camphor, and limonene, all have antiseptic effects.

☞ DIRECTIONS: Crush some chaparral leaves. (You can use fresh leaves if you live in the Southwest and can find them.) Mix the leaves with an equal amount of lard and simmer the mixture on the lowest possible heat for two to three hours. Strain and allow the salve to cool to room temperature. Apply to sores three to four times a day for as long as desired.

YERBA MANSA: Among American Indians and Hispanic settlers, yerba mansa (*Anemopsis californica*) was the most popular medicinal herb of traditional medicine in the Southwest. Spanish settlers learned the plant's uses from the Maricopa, Pima, Tewa, and Yaqui Indian tribes. "Yerba mansa" is short for "yerba del indio manso," or "herb of the tamed Indians."

The plant was used both externally and internally to treat a variety of conditions, especially those affecting the mucous membranes. It may be best suited to treat ulcerations of the mouth or lips. Yerba mansa contains the volatile constituents thymol and methyl eugenol, both of which have demonstrated antimicrobial properties. Its use was adopted by the Eclectic physicians in 1877.

☞ DIRECTIONS: Place 1 ounce of yerba mansa in 1 pint of water, bring to a boil, and simmer for twenty to thirty minutes. Let stand until cool. Apply the tea to the ulcer every few hours with a clean cloth. Continue doing this as long as desired.

ALOE VERA: Although aloe vera is better known, as a burn remedy, the Amish also use it to treat sores and ulcers. Aloe vera, in addition to its ability to reduce pain and inflammation, also has antiseptic effects that make it useful for treating infected ulcers. In 1988 at the University of Puerto Rico, during research on the plant's effects on burns, it was discovered that not only did aloe vera gel speed the healing time of burns but it also reduced the bacterial counts in the burns. We can suppose that it has the same effect on skin ulcers.

☞ DIRECTIONS: Break off a piece of an aloe vera leaf. Apply the juicy sap to the skin ulcer. You can also purchase some aloe vera gel at a health food store and use that instead of the plant's sap. Repeat the applications every few hours. Continue doing this as long as desired.

PLANTAIN LEAVES: Plantain (Plantago major) is a common lawn weed throughout North America. Although it arrived in North America with the English colonists, its use was rapidly adopted by the indigenous residents of the continent. The Delaware, Mohegan, Ojibwa, Cherokee, and many other Indian tribes have used plantain to disinfect and relieve the symptoms of minor wounds and other skin conditions. The plant contains a large number of anti-inflammatory constituents and at least six antiseptic ones. Plantain also contains the constituent allantoin, which promotes cell proliferation and tissue healing. Fresh leaves must be used to derive the antiseptic benefits.

☞ DIRECTIONS: Crush a small handful of fresh plantain leaves and apply the juice to the ulcer. Hold the leaves in place against the ulcer with a bandage. Renew the dressing three to four times a day. Continue doing this as long as desired.

PINE AND PINE BARK: Pine bark poultices *(Pinus spp.)* appear in the folklore of a number of American Indian tribes for treating sores. The practice, whether it was introduced by the Indians or borrowed from similar traditions in Europe, was later adopted by the colonists. The remedy is still practiced today in the folklore of North Carolina and Appalachia. Pine sap contains a variety of antimicrobial substances.

☞ DIRECTIONS: Strip some bark from the branches of a white pine. Boil the bark in water for twenty to thirty minutes. Let cool. Then scrape the soft inner bark away from the hard outer bark. Moisten with liquor to make a poultice and apply to sores three to four times a day.

Alternately, purchase some White Pine Compound Syrup, a nonprescription item, at a pharmacy. Apply to the ulcer with a clean cloth three to four times a day. Be careful not to irritate the skin with the pine syrup.

ROSEMARY: A remedy for sores from the Hispanic folklore of the Southwest is rosemary leaf *(Rosmarinus officinalis)*. Rosemary contains more than ten antiseptic constituents.

☞ DIRECTIONS: Crush some rosemary leaves and

mix with an equal amount of hot honey. Keep the mixture warm on a hot plate or in a crock pot for half an hour. Using gauze, apply to the ulcer and use a bandage to hold the mixture in place. Change the dressing two to three times a day. Alternately, place 1 ounce of rosemary leaf in a 1-pint jar and fill with boiling water. Cover tightly and let stand until the water reaches room temperature. Strain. Apply the solution to the ulcers every hour or two, using a clean cloth.

GINGER POULTICE: A collection of remedies, called *American Folk Medicine,* lists an 1831 entry calling for a poultice of ginger (*Zingiber officinalis*) and slippery elm (*Ulmus fulva*) to treat sores. The slippery elm is mucilaginous and forms the bulk of the poultice. The spicy oils in ginger are antibacterial and also stimulate local circulation to the skin.

☞ DIRECTIONS: Boil ½ cup of water and add 1 tablespoon of ginger powder. Allow to steep for a minute or two, and then stir in slippery elm powder until a thick mass forms. Allow to cool. Apply enough of the mixture to cover the ulcer, and hold it in place with gauze and a bandage. Change the dressing two to three times a day. Continue using this remedy for as long as desired.

ONION: In the folk medicine of Appalachia and the Southwest, onion poultices (*Allium cepa*) are used to treat sores and ulcers. Onion, like garlic, contains antibacterial compounds, including allicin, which is also in garlic. Onion is not as irritating to the skin as garlic and it is less likely to cause skin burns. Its mild irritation, in addition to its killing microorganisms, increases local circulation.

☞ DIRECTIONS: Pulverize half an onion in a blender, or crush until juicy with a mortar and pestle. Mix the onion with a little honey and apply to the ulcer. Don't leave in place for more than an hour. Then wash the ulcer and cover with a clean dressing. Do this three times a day. Don't use this treatment on patients with paralysis or other conditions that would prevent them from feeling any irritation that might be caused by the onion salve.

CALENDULA: British folk medicine records the saying "Where there is calendula, there is no need of a surgeon." But calendula (Calendula officinalis) is not really a miracle herb that can prevent modern surgery. The British saying was coined during a time when the most common surgery was amputation and the most common cause of amputation was infected wounds.

Calendula has been used to cleanse wounds and promote healing since ancient times. The plant's flowers contain constituents that kill bacteria, viruses, and molds, as well as other constituents that are powerfully anti-inflammatory. Still more constituents promote cell growth in wounds and ulcers. Calendula is approved in Germany today in topical preparations that are specifically designed to treat ulcers and slow-healing wounds.

A caution with calendula: Do not use it on wounds or ulcers that are oozing pus. The plant can promote cell growth so efficiently that it can cause a wound to close prematurely and form an abscess, raising the risk of systemic infection. Calendula, which is also called "pot marigold," is a different plant than the common garden marigold (Tagetes erecta), which contains different constituents than calendula.

☞ DIRECTIONS: Place 1 ounce of calendula flowers in a 1-pint jar and fill with boiling water. Cover the jar tightly and allow to steep until the brew reaches room temperature. Strain. Apply externally with a clean cloth to ulcers and slow-healing wounds. Allow the area to dry and then place a dressing on the sore. Reapply three to four times a day. Also, take 1 tablespoon of the tea internally along with each external application.

Alternately, crush several handfuls of dried calendula flowers into a powder and place in a crock pot or glass pot on a hot plate. Add enough honey to cover. Allow to steep on the lowest heat for ten to fifteen minutes after the honey has melted. Let cool to room temperature. Do not strain. Apply with gauze to the wound and use a bandage to hold the gauze in place. Apply three to four times a day. Remember to clean the wound well each time to remove any plant material or honey before reapplying the remedy.

GUMWEED: Gumweed *(Grindelia spp.)* is a major skin remedy of the American Indians of the Southwest and northwestern Mexico. The plant entered into Eclectic medical practice during the late 19th century. Eclectic professor Harvey Felter, M.D., stated in *The Eclectic Materia Medica, Pharmacology, and Therapeutics* that gumweed was especially well suited to skin conditions with poor circulation and a tendency to form ulcers. Gumweed was an official medicine in the *United States Pharmacopoeia* from 1882 until 1926. The plant's resin contains anti-inflammatory and antimicrobial constituents.

☞ DIRECTIONS: Apply the sticky sap from the leaves or flowers of gumweed to the affected areas. Reapply every few hours. Cover with gauze and a clean bandage. Alternately, you can purchase some tincture of gumweed, and use it as a wash. Reapply every few hours.

GYPSY SALVE: A Gypsy salve for ulcers and poorly healing wounds combines a number of the other remedies mentioned in this section. The Spanish Gypsy herbalist Pilar, who provided the remedies published in the book *Gypsy Folk Medicine* by folklorist Wanja von Hausen, calls the ointment "Bride of the Sun Salve." The remedy is slightly modified below for ease of use.

☞ DIRECTIONS: Warm 1 cup of olive oil in a pan. Mix a handful of pot marigold flowers *(Calendula officinalis),* 9 rosemary blossoms, and 9 lavender blossoms into the oil. Simmer for three minutes, and remove from heat. Pulverize 3 cloves of garlic (not the larger bulbs) in a blender or use a mortar and pestle. Add the garlic to the oil. Let cool to room temperature, cover, and store overnight. Heat the salve again the next day on the lowest possible heat for seven minutes. Let cool to room temperature. Strain the mixture and apply to the wound. Reapply three to four times a day as often as desired.

❧ Splinters ❧

Splinters under the skin are a common occurrence wherever people live or work. They were probably even more common in the past, when our ancestors used more wooden implements and worked with more rough and unfinished wood than we do today. We still get splinters, however, and they are still sometimes hard to get out.

The best method to extract a splinter is to use a pair of tweezers. Pull the splinter out gently, taking care not to leave any broken pieces behind. Then clean the wound thoroughly to prevent infection. Application of topical anti-infectives (alcohol or an antibiotic ointment) are recommended.

The folk remedies for extracting splinters and thorns generally act to soften or moisten the area around the sliver or to "draw" the object to the surface for easier extraction with the fingers or with tweezers.

A deep splinter may require the assistance of a physician, who can use surgical instruments to remove it and can give antibiotics to prevent infection. Even modern medical treatment for splinters sometimes fails, however, because the imbedded pieces of the splinter are not visible on X ray unless they are metallic.

The chief health risk of splinters, especially those that go deep into the tissues, is tetanus, or lockjaw. In this disease, a germ that is common in animal feces, and in soil that has been exposed to animal feces, infects the wound. The germ produces a nerve toxin that can result in death. Tetanus is a rare disease in North America. In the 1990s, fewer than a hundred cases a year have been reported. Nevertheless, it is a serious illness, with about a 50 percent mortality rate, so a tetanus shot is prudent, especially if a splinter or other wound goes deep into the tissues and carries dirt with it.

Remedies

PLANTAIN LEAVES: Plantain (*Plantago major*) has been used in cultures around the world as a drawing and wound-healing agent. Applied externally, the plant stimulates and cleanses the skin and encourages wounds to
continued on page 365

Studying the Calendar

⊠ ⊠ ⊠

Time is a critical element in many folk medical practices. Certain days, months, or seasons of the year were said to be the best—or worst—time to take or make medicine, to get sick, or to get well.

> *January will search,*
> *February will try,*
> *March will tell if you'll*
> *live or die.*

A spring tonic was taken to "clean the blood" after the long winter. The great variety of teas and formulas used for this purpose attest to the widespread desire to "open the system and clean it out" and "pep it up." An Ohio farmer in the 1950s said he sold thousands of bunches of red sassafras for tonic each spring. He dug up the plants in the dark of the moon in February when they were supposed to be "full of the vitamins and minerals for a healthy life."

Some calendrical ideas and practices have an obvious basis in fact, while others are based on outmoded ideas about nature or the body. Winter is, of course, the riskiest season for influenza and other diseases that spread in close quarters, so there is reason in the rhyme above. But the idea that the blood needs "purifying," or that this can be done with laxatives (which is what many "tonics" were) is rejected by medical science. Despite this, digging sassafras root in February might—or might not—be done because it is believed the active compounds are most concentrated then. Many medicinal plants are supposed to be harvested at certain times of the day or year in order to be effective as medicine, so they well may have the desired properties only at a certain season or state of maturity.

Sometimes it seems easy to separate "magic" from "material" medicine: The leaves or bark of a tree to be used for an emetic (a vomit inducer), for instance, is supposed to be stripped upwards. If it is to be used for a laxative, it is stripped downwards. Because the direction in which the leaves are stripped could not really reverse their medicinal effect, this is a magical cure even though it uses plant medicine. But say an herb is to be picked only on Saint John's Day. This remedy sounds more like "magic," but perhaps midsummer is when the herb is actually the most potent, and fixing that day merely encoded that fact.

One of the major shapers of American folk medicine, the almanac, influenced many time-related beliefs. Throughout the 16th and 17th centuries, these how-to guides were the only book other than the Bible in many households. Almanacs contained thousands of "receipts," or recipes, for cures. A perennial feature of the earlier almanacs was the "Man of the Signs"—a human figure surrounded by astrological signs designating various parts of his anatomy. The reader consulted tables inside as to the best time for attention to these parts. Well into the 20th century people spoke of remedies to be undertaken (or avoided) when "the sign is in the head" or "in the knees." The almanacs also gave health hints for each month. The readers of *Poor Robin's Almanac* for 1728 were given this advice for November:

"The best Physick in this month is good Exercise, warmth, and wholesome Meat and Drink. Kill your swine in this Month, and after Pork and Pease be sure to break Wind."

Phases of the moon have been thought to affect the body, especially the full moon, which was supposed to make sick people sicker. People having surgery during a full moon would bleed more. Light shining on the face of a healthy person while he slept could drain him of his strength. On the other hand, medicine taken during this time was especially effective because the sickness would decrease along with the moon. The principle was similar to planting crops, brewing, or butchering by the moon: Waxing and fullness fostered growth; waning produced the opposite. You could thus plant potatoes by the full moon for a healthy family.

The most patently magical health customs are the once-a-year observances to insure health for the rest of the year: Walk barefoot in the first snow and wash in the first May rain. New Year's Day is naturally favored for the practicing of customs, so you should wipe down all the doorknobs at the stroke of twelve on this day for better health. Holidays are common occasions for such magical actions, and sometimes religious symbolism from the church is carried over into the home. Catholics would put blessed palms from Palm Sunday on the walls of their houses or hang bouquets blessed on the Assumption. Other symbolic rites had a completely secular, spell-like character. You could eat the first fresh fruit of the season and say, "First fruit into my stomach, illness to hell." You could throw an apple, cake, and salt into the well on Christmas Eve and say, "Cold water, I am giving you these gifts, now you give me health and happiness." The most common annual health-bringing act was merely to eat a special food on a special day, like goose for Christmas and hog's head on New Year's.

A time for every purpose under heaven.

Marking the calendar with health-related customs affirmed the importance of health in the cycles of life.

heal faster. It was naturalized in North America
after the arrival of the
Europeans, and American
Indians called it "White
Man's Foot-print," because
it seemed to follow the
European colonists wher-
ever they went. The
Delaware, Mohegan,
Ojibwa, Cherokee, and
many other Indian tribes
used plantain to treat minor
wounds and insect bites.
Hardy and adaptable,
plantain has made itself at
home throughout the world.
Often you'll see it growing
along roads, in meadows,
and, to the chagrin of
homeowners, in lawns.

☞ DIRECTIONS: Crush
up plantain leaves and
apply them directly to the
wound.

BREAD AND WATER: In
New England folk
medicine a

Pork

Farmers throughout the
eastern and midwestern
United States have applied
pork or bacon poultices to
the skin to draw out splinters. Why pork? Probably
because of its salt, which
acts as an astringent. (Pork
and bacon have tradition-
ally been cured in salt.)
You might improve on the
method and avoid some of
the mess by soaking the
injured area in hot salt
water until you can better
get at the splinter with a
pair of tweezers.

poultice of bread and
water or bread and milk
is a favorite for treating
splinters. In *Country Folk
Remedies: Tales of Skunk
Oil, Sassafras Tea and
Other Old-Time
Remedies Gathered
by Elisabeth Janos,*
one elderly New
England gen-
tleman once said
that he would refuse
to eat bread pudding

when he was growing up because he was afraid he would be eating a poultice. The combination of heat and the astringent action of the drying bread combine to soften the skin and draw the splinter out.

☞ DIRECTIONS: Break up the bread and mix it with milk or water. Heat the mixture on the stove and apply it as hot as you can tolerate. Let it cool on the wound in order to bring the splinter closer to the surface of the skin.

SUGAR AND SOAP: Early Indiana settlers used a mixture of sugar and soap. This poultice combines both moistening and drawing qualities.

☞ DIRECTIONS: Mix equal parts of brown sugar and laundry soap. Moisten and apply to the wound for up to twenty-four hours.

SUCTION: Using suction is a traditional New England method for drawing out splinters. This method is closely related to "cupping," a practice that remains a part of tradi-

tional medicine throughout Europe, the Middle East, and Asia.

☞ DIRECTIONS: Fill a wide-mouthed bottle with steaming hot water. Put the injured spot over the mouth of the bottle and press down. As the steam cools, it quickly forms a suction, drawing the skin lightly up into the jar. The steam softens the tissues and the suction will stretch the skin and draw the splinter to the surface.

CLAY PACKS: Clay or mud packs were favorite wound-healing and splinter-extracting poultices used by various American Indian groups as well as the German immigrants of the 18th century. Any type of clean clay soil (free from animal fecal matter or other pollutants) will do.

☞ DIRECTIONS: Make a poultice by mixing the clay with hot water. Apply to the wound. Let the mixture dry, then flake the residue off. If the splinter still isn't close enough to the surface to draw it out, apply another poultice.

❦ Bibliography ❦

Books and Periodicals

Baldwin, Rahima. *Special Delivery.* Berkeley, California: Celestial Arts, 1979.

Bell, Whitfield J. *The Colonial Physician and Other Essays.* New York: Science History Publications, 1975.

Bhagvan-Dash, Vaidya. *Materia Medica of Ayurveda.* New Delhi: B. Jain Publishers, 1991.

Boyle, Wade. *Herb Doctors: Pioneers in 19th-Century American Botanical Medicine and a History of the Eclectic Medical Institute of Cincinnati.* East Palestine, Ohio: Buckeye Naturopathic Press, 1988.

Boyle, Wade. *Official Herbs: Botanical Substances in the United States Pharmacopoeias, 1820-1990.* East Palestine, Ohio: Buckeye Naturopathic Press, 1991.

Cameron, M.L. *Anglo-Saxon Medicine.* Cambridge, England: Cambridge University Press, 1993.

Casetta, Anna; Hand, Wayland D.; and Pickett, Newbell Niles. *Popular Beliefs and Superstitions: A Compendium of American Folklore.* Boston: G.K. Hall, 1981, 3 volumes. (Copyright: John G. White Department of the Cleveland Public Library, 1981.)

Castetter, Edward F., and Ruth M. Underhill. "The Ethnobiology of the Papago Indians: Ethnobiological Studies in the American Southwest." *The University of New Mexico Bulletin* #275, Vol. II, 1935.

Chevallier, Andrew. *The Encyclopedia of Medicinal Plants.* New York: DK Publishing, 1996.

Chishti, Hakim G.M. *The Traditional Healer: A Comprehensive Guide to the Principles and Practice of Unani Herbal Medicine.* Rochester, Vermont: Inner Traditions International Ltd., 1988.

Classen, Constance; Howes, David; and Synnott, Anthony. *Aroma: The Cultural History of Smell.* London and New York: Routledge, 1994.

Colby, Benjamin. *A Guide to Health, Being an Exposition of the Principles of the Thomsonian System of Practice, and Their Mode of Application in the Cure of Every Form of Disease,* 3rd ed. Milford, New Hampshire: John Burns, 1846.

Cook, William H. *The Physio-Medicalist Dispensatory.* Cincinnati, Ohio: Wm. H. Cook, 1869.

Crellin, John K., and Jane Philpott. *Herbal Medicine Past and Present: Trying to Give Ease.* (Vol. I) Durham, North Carolina: Duke University Press, 1997.

Crellin, John K., and Jane Philpott. *Herbal Medicine Past and Present: A Reference Guide to Medicinal Plants.* (Vol. II) Durham, North Carolina: Duke University Press, 1997.

Culpeper, Nicholas. *Culpeper's Complete Herbal: Consisting of a Comprehensive Description of Nearly All Herbs With Their Medicinal Properties and Directions for Compounding the Medicines Extracted From Them.* London, England: Foulsham & Company Ltd., 1995.

Densmore, Frances. "Uses of Plants by the Chippewa Indians." *SI-BAE Annual Report* (1928), pp. 44: 273-379.

Der Marderosian, Ara, and Lawrence E. Liberti. *Natural Product Medicine: A Scientific Guide to Foods, Drugs, Cosmetics.* Philadelphia, Pennsylvania: Lippincott-Raven Publishers, 1988.

Edelsward, L.M. *Sauna as Symbol: Society and Culture in Finland.* New York: Peter Lang, 1991.

Ellingwood, Finley. *American Materia, Therapeutics and Pharmacology.* Portland, Oregon: Eclectic Medical Publications, 1919.

Erichsen-Brown, Charlotte. *Medicinal and other Uses of North American Plants: A Historical Survey with Special Reference to the Eastern Indian Tribes.* New York: Dover Publications, 1979.

Felter, Harvey. *The Eclectic Materia Medica, Pharmacology, and Therapeutics.* Portland, Oregon: Eclectic Medical Publications, 1922.

Felter, Harvey, and John U. Lloyd. *King's American Dispensatory,* Vol. I and II. Portland, Oregon: Eclectic Medical Publications, 1898.

Ferreira, Antonio. *Prenatal Environment.* Springfield, Illinois: Charles C. Thomas, 1969.

Firestone, Melvin M. "Sephardic Folk-Curing in Seattle." *Journal of American Folklore,* Vol. 75 (1962), pp. 301-310.

Fontenot, Wonda L. *Secret Doctors: Ethnomedicine of African Americans.* Westport, Connecticut: Bergin and Garvey, 1994.

Frankel, Barbara. *Childbirth in the Ghetto: Folk Beliefs of Negro Women in a North Philadelphia Hospital Ward.* San Francisco: R & E Research Associates, 1977.

Fried, Lewis. *Handbook of American-Jewish Literature: An Analytic Guide to Topics, Themes, and Sources.* New York: Greenwood Press, 1988.

Gilmore, Melvin R. *Some Chippewa Uses of Plants.* Ann Arbor, Michigan: University of Michigan Press, 1933.

Grieve, M. *A Modern Herbal,* Vol. I and II. New York: Dover Publications, 1978.

Grinnell, George Bird. *The Cheyenne Indians: Their History and Ways of Life,* Vol. II. Lincoln, Nebraska: University of Nebraska Press, 1972.

Grünwald, Jörg. Heilpflanzen: *Herbal Remedies.* (CD-ROM) Berlin: Thomas Brendler, 1996.

Halpert, Herbert. "Supernatural Sanctions and the Legend." *Folklore Studies in the Twentieth Century*, ed. V. Newall, Woodbridge, U.K.: D.S. Brewer, 1978.

Hamel, Paul B., and M.U. Chiltoskey. *Cherokee Plants*. Sylva, North Carolina: Herald Pub. Co., 1975.

Hand, Wayland. *American Folk Medicine: A Symposium*. Berkeley and Los Angeles, California: University of California Press, 1976.

Hand, Wayland. *Magical Medicine: The Folkloric Component of Medicine in the Folk Belief, Custom, and Ritual of the Peoples of Europe and America*. Berkeley and Los Angeles, California: University of California Press, 1980.

Hand, Wayland, ed. *The Frank C. Brown Collection of North Carolina Folklore, Vol. VI, Popular Beliefs and Superstitions from North Carolina*. Durham, North Carolina: Duke University Press, 1961.

Harding, A.R. *Ginseng and Other Medicinal Plants*, revised ed. Columbus, Ohio: A.R. Harding, 1972.

Harris, Marvin. *Culture, Man, and Nature: An Introduction to General Anthropology*. New York: Thomas Y. Crowell Company, 1971.

Hatfield, Gabrielle. *Country Remedies: Traditional East Anglian Plant Remedies in the Twentieth Century*. Woodbridge, Suffolk: Colleagues Press, 1995.

Hendrickson, Robert. *The Facts on File Encyclopedia of Word and Phrase Origins*. New York and Oxford: Facts on File Publications, 1987.

Herrick, James W., and Dean R. Snow. *Iroquois Medical Botany*. Syracuse, New York: Syracuse University Press, 1994.

Hister, Art. *Dr. Art Hister's Do-It-Yourself Guide to Good Health*. Toronto, Canada: Random House, 1978.

Hoebel, E. Adamson. *The Cheyennes: Indians of the Great Plains*. New York: Holt, Rinehart and Winston, 1960.

Hsu, Hong-Yen. *Oriental Materia Medica: A Concise Guide*. New Canaan, Connecticut: Keats Publishing, 1986.

Hufford, David J. "Contemporary Folk Medicine." *In Other Healers: Unorthodox Medicine in America*, ed. Norman Gevitz. Baltimore: Johns Hopkins University Press, 1988, pp. 228-264.

Hunter, David E. and Phillip Whitten, ed. *Encyclopedia of Anthropology*. New York: Harper-Collins, 1976.

Hyatt, Harry M. *Hoodoo—Conjuration—Witchcraft—Rootwork*. Hannibal, Missouri: Western Publising Company, 1970, 4 volumes.

Janos, Elisabeth. *Country Folk Remedies: Tales of Skunk Oil, Sassafras Tea and Other Old-Time Remedies Gathered by Elisabeth Janos*. New York: Galahad Books, 1990.

Jarvis, D.C. *Folk Remedies: A Vermont Doctor's Guide to Good Health.* New York: Holt, Rinehart, and Winston, 1958.

Kelly, Isabel. *Folk Practices in North Mexico: Birth Customs, Folk Medicine, and Spiritualism in the Laguna Zone.* Austin, Texas: Institute of Latin American Studies, University of Texas Press, 1965.

Kingston, Maxine Hong. *The Woman Warrior: Memoirs of a Girlhood Among Ghosts.* New York: Vintage, 1989.

Kirchfeld, Friedhelm, and Wade Boyle. *Nature Doctors: Pioneers in Naturopathic Medicine.* Portland, Oregon: Medicina Biologica, 1994.

Kitzinger, Sheila; Jessel, Camilla; and Nancy Durrell McKenna. *The Complete Book of Pregnancy and Childbirth.* New York: Alfred A. Knopf, 1991.

Kneipp, Sebastian. *My Water Cure.* New York: Mokelumne Hill Press, 1972.

Krochmal, Arnold and Connie. *A Guide to the Medicinal Plants of the U.S.* New York: Quadrangle, 1973.

Krupat, Arnold. *For Those Who Came After: A Study of Native American Autobiography.* Chicago: University of Chicago Press, 1989.

Ladenheim, Melissa. *The Sauna in Central New York.* Ithaca, New York: DeWitt Historical Society, 1986.

Laguerre, Michel. *Afro-Caribbean Folk Medicine.* South Hadley, Massachusetts: Bergin and Garvey, 1988.

Latham, Minor White. *The Elizabethan Fairies: The Fairies of Folklore and the Fairies of Shakespeare,* 1930. (Reprint New York: Octagon, 1972.)

Leslie, Charles M., ed. *Asian Medical Systems: A Comparitive Study.* Berkeley, California: University of California Press, 1976.

Leung, Albert Y. *Chinese Herbal Remedies.* New York: Universe, 1984.

Lewis, Walter H., et al. *Medical Botany: Plants Affecting Man's Health.* New York: John Wiley & Sons, 1982.

Lindlahr, Henry. *Natural Therapeutics,* Vol. II. Saffron Walden, United Kingdom: C.W. Daniel Company, 1983.

Logan, Patrick. *Making the Cure: A Look at Irish Folk Medicine.* Dublin, Ireland: The Talbot Press, 1975.

Malpezzi, Frances M. and William M. Clements. *Italian-American Folklore.* Little Rock, Arkansas: August House Publishers, 1992.

Manniche, Lise. *An Ancient Egyptian Herbal.* Austin, Texas: University of Texas Press, 1989.

Maressa, John. *Maqiuq: The Eskimo Sweat Bath.* Hohenschaftlarn: Klaus Renner, 1986.

McBride, L.R. *Practical Folk Medicine of Hawaii.* Hilo, Hawaii: The Petroglyph Press, 1975.

McGrath, William R. *Amish Folk Remedies for Plain and Fancy Ailments.* Burr Oak, Michigan: Schupps Herbs & Vitamins, 1987.

McGuffin, Michael; Hobbs, Christopher; Upton, Roy; and Goldberg, Alicia. *American Herbal Products Association's Botanical Safety Handbook.* Boca Raton, Florida: CRC Press, 1997.

McIntyre, Anne. *Folk Remedies for Common Ailments.* Toronto, Ontario: Key Porter Books Ltd., 1994.

McMahon, William. *Pine Barrens Legends, Lore and Lies.* Wilmington, Delaware: Middle Atlantic Press, 1980.

Meyer, Clarence. *American Folk Medicine.* New York: Meyerbooks, 1985.

Meyer, George G. *Folk Medicine and Herbal Healing.* Springfield, Illinois: Charles C. Thomas, 1981.

Milinaire, Caterine. *Birth: Facts and Legends.* New York: Harmony Books, 1974.

Moerman, Daniel E. *Geraniums for the Iroquois: A Field Guide to American Indian Medicinal Plants.* Algonac, Michigan: Reference Publications, Inc., 1982.

Moore, Michael. *Medicinal Plants of the Mountain West.* Santa Fe, New Mexico: Museum of New Mexico Press, 1979.

Moore, Michael. *Medicinal Plants of the Desert and Canyon West.* Santa Fe, New Mexico: Museum of New Mexico Press, 1989.

Moore, Michael and Mimi Kamp. *Los Remedios: Traditional Herbal Remedies of the Southwest.* Santa Fe, New Mexico: Red Crane Books, 1990.

Naeser, Margaret A. *Outline Guide to Chinese Herbal Patent Medicines in Pill Form: An Introduction to Chinese Herbal Medicines.* Boston, Massachusetts: Boston Chinese Medicine, 1990.

Nagy, Doreen Evenden. *Popular Medicine in Seventeenth-Century England.* Bowling Green, Ohio: Bowling Green State University Popular Press, 1988.

Newall, Carol et al. *Herbal Medicines: A Guide for Health Care Professionals.* London, England: Rittenhouse Book Distributors, 1996.

O'Connor, Bonnie Blair. *Healing Traditions: Alternative Medicine and the Health Professions.* Philadelphia, Pennsylvania: University of Pennsylvania Press, 1995.

Ody, Penelope. *The Complete Medical Herbal.* London: Key Porter Books, 1994.

Opie, Iona and Moira Tatem, eds. *A Dictionary of Superstitions.* Oxford, England: Oxford University Press, 1989.

Osol, Arthur, and George E. Farrar. *The Dispensatory of the United States of America,* 24th ed. Philadelphia, Pennsylvania: J.B. Lippencott Company, 1947.

Patai, Raphael. *On Jewish Folklore.* Detroit, Michigan: Wayne State University Press, 1983.

Pedersen, Mark. *Nutritional Herbology: A Reference Guide to Herbs.* Warsaw, Indiana: Wendell W. Whitman Company, 1994.

Rafinesque, C. *Medical Flora: Manual of the Medical Botany of the United States,* Vol. II. Philadelphia, Pennsylvania: Samuel C. Atkinson, 1830.

Ray, Verne F. "The Sanpoil and Nespelem: Salishan Peoples of N.E. Washington." *University of Washington Publications in Anthropology,* Vol. V, 1933.

Roeder, Beatrice A. *Chicano Folk Medicine from Los Angeles, California.* Berkeley, California: University of California Press, 1988.

Root-Bernstein, Robert S., and Michéle Root-Bernstein. *Honey, Mud, Maggots, and Other Medical Marvels: The Science Behind Folk Remedies and Old Wives' Tales.* Boston, Massachusetts: Houghton Mifflin, 1997.

Rorie, David. *Folk Tradition and Folk Medicine in Scotland: The Writings of David Rorie,* ed. David Buchan. Edinburgh, Scotland: Canongate Academic, 1994.

Sagendorph, Robb. *America and her Almanacs: Wit, Wisdom & Weather.* Brown, Massachusetts: Little, Brown, 1970.

Samuels, Mike, and Nancy Samuels. *The Well Pregnancy Book.* New York: Summit Books, 1986.

Saxon, Lyle. *Gumbo Ya-Ya: Folk Tales of Louisiana.* Boston, Massachusetts: Houghton Mifflin, 1945.

Shyrock, Richard Harris. *Medicine in America: Historical Essays.* Baltimore, Maryland: The Johns Hopkins Press, 1966.

Slater, Candace. *Dance of the Dolphin: Transformation and Disenchantment in the Amazonian Imagination.* Chicago: University of Chicago Press, 1994.

Smith, Huron H. "Ethnobotany of the Ojibwa Indians." *Bulletin of the Public Museum of Milwaukee* (1932), pp. 4: 327-525.

Snow, Loudell F. *Walkin' Over Medicine.* Boulder, Colorado: Westview Press, 1993.

Speck, Frank G. "Catawba Medicines and Curative Practices." *Publications of the Philadelphia Anthropological Society,* Vol. I, 1937.

Spicer, Edward H. and Eleanor Bauwens. *Ethnic Medicine in the Southwest.* Tucson, Arizona: University of Arizona Press, 1977.

Steedman, E.V. "The Ethnobotany of the Thompson Indians." *SI-BAE Annual Report* (1928), pp. 45: 441-522.

Stone, Eric. *Medicine Among the American Indians.* New York: Hafner Publishing, 1962.

Stowell, Marion Barber. *Early American Almanacs: The Colonial Weekday Bible.* New York: Lenox Hill Publishers, 1977.

Strehlow, Wighard and Gottfried Hertzka. *Hildegarde of Bingen's Medicine.* Santa Fe, New Mexico: Bear and Company, 1988.

Tantaquidgeon, Gladys. *A Study of Delaware Indian Medicine Practice and Folk Beliefs.* Harrisburg, Pennsylvania: Pennsylvania Historical Commission, 1942.

Terrell, Suzanne J. *This Other Kind of Doctors: Traditional Medical Systems in Black Neighborhoods in Austin, Texas.* New York: AMS Press, 1990.

Thomson, Samuel. "A Narrative of the Life & Medical Discoveries of Samuel Thomson, Containing an Account of His System and the Manner of Curing." *Twelve Works of Naive Genius,* ed. Walter Teller. Ayer Co. Pub., 1972, pp. 17-60.

Thrash, Agatha, and Calvin Thrash. *Home Remedies: Hydrotherapy, Massage, Charcoal, and Other Simple Treatments.* Seale, Alabama: Newlifestyle Books, 1981.

Trachtenberg, Joshua. *Jewish Magic and Superstition: A Study in Folk Religion,* 1939. (Reprint New York: Atheneum, 1970.)

Trotter, Robert T. *Curanderismo: Mexican-American Folk Healing.* Second Edition. Athens, Georgia: University of Georgia Press, 1997.

Tyler, Varro. *Herbs of Choice: The Therapeutic Use of Phytomedicinals.* New York: Haworth Press, 1994.

Tyler, Varro. *Hoosier Home Remedies.* West Lafayette, Indiana: Purdue University Press, 1985.

Tyler, Varro. *The Honest Herbal: A Sensible Guide to the Use of Herbs and Related Remedies.* Third Edition. New York: Haworth Press, 1993.

Val Alphen, Jan and Anthony Aris, ed. *Oriental Medicine: An Illustrated Guide to the Asian Arts of Healing.* Boston: Shambhala, 1996.

Vance, Randolph. *Ozark Magic and Folklore,* 1947. (Reprint New York: Dover, 1964.)

Vogel, Virgil. *American Indian Medicine.* Norman, Oklahoma: University of Oklahoma Press, 1970.

von Hausen, Wanja. *Gypsy Folk Medicine.* New York: Sterling Publishing Company, 1992.

Weiss, Rudolf Fritz. *Herbal Medicine.* Beaconsfield, England: Beaconsfield Publishers, 1988. (Translated from: *Lehrbuch der Phytotherapie,* 6th ed. Stuttgart: Hippokrates Verlag, 1985.)

Williams, Phyllis H. *South Italian Folkways in Europe and America.* New Haven, Connecticut: Yale University Press, 1938.

Wood, Matthew. *The Magical Staff: Handing Down the Tradition of Natural Medicine.* Berkeley, California: North Atlantic Books, 1992.

Woodward, Marcus, ed. *Gerard's Herbal.* London, England: Studio Editions, 1994.

Yoffie, Leah Rachel. "Popular Beliefs and Customs among the Yiddish-Speaking Jews of St. Louis, Mo." *Journal of American Folklore,* Vol. 38 (1925), pp. 375-399.

Young, James Harvey. *The Toadstool Millionaires: A Social History of Patent Medicines in America Before Federal Regulation.* Princeton: Princeton University Press, 1961.

❦ Index ❧

■ ■ ■